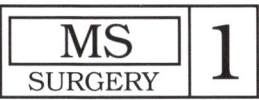 **Master Series in Surgery**

Series Editor:
Dana K. Andersen, MD

Brought to you as an educational service by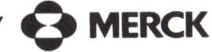

Advance *noun*....progress, improvement, movement toward a goal.

Each volume in the Master Series in Surgery *will provide a comprehensive review of current advances in a major area of surgery. The objective is to provide the reader with practical, up-to-date information and to favor the clinical more than the experimental aspect of the topics presented. However, special attention will be devoted to the discussion of recent investigative findings that might impact the conduct of surgical and clinical practices in these areas. The volumes of the series are not intended to serve as "how-to" books, but as useful references by authorities in the field.*

Series Editor: Dana K. Andersen, MD

Forthcoming Volumes:

Volume 2 Advances in Surgery in the Elderly
Volume 3 Advances in Colorectal Carcinoma Surgery
Volume 4 Advances in Wound Healing and Tissue Repair

Advances in Minimally Invasive Surgery

Volume 1
Master Series in Surgery

Series Editor: Dana K. Andersen, MD
Professor of Surgery and Medicine
Chief, Section of General Surgery
Department of Surgery
The University of Chicago

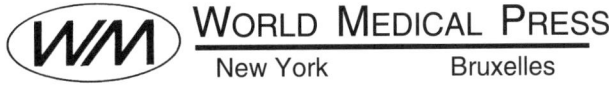

Library of Congress Cataloging in Publication Data
Main entry under title:
Advances in Minimally Invasive Surgery
(Master Series in Surgery)
Includes bibliographies and index.

© 1993 World Medical Press
Division, World Medical Communications Organization, Inc.

All rights reserved. No part of this book may be translated or reproduced in any form without written permission from World Medical Press, 7 Ridgedale Avenue, Cedar Knolls, New Jersey 07927, USA. The use of general descriptive names, trade names, trademarks, etc, in this publication, even if the former are not especially identified, is not to be taken as a sign that such names, as understood by the Trade Marks and Merchanise Marks Act, may accordingly be used freely by anyone. While the advice and information in this book is believed to be true and accurate at the date of going to press, neither the authors nor the editors nor the publisher can accept any legal responsibility for any errors or omissions that may be made. The publisher makes no warranty, express or implied, with respect to the material contained herein. The reader is urged to review the package information data of the manufacturers of the devices and/or medications mentioned.

Printed in the United States of America

ISBN 0-933751-02-8 World Medical Press   New York/Bruxelles

Preface

TO THE SERIES

Our goal in this and future volumes of the *Master Series in Surgery* is to provide the general surgeon with the best information available regarding the understanding and management of clinical disorders. Our contributors have been selected because of their ability to translate the latest observations in their field to clearly defined principles of surgical care. Topics of future monographs have been selected to focus on areas in which new developments have begun to impact on patient care. The rapid publication format of this series is designed to update the reader to the newest aspects of important problems in general surgery.

TO VOLUME 1

Laparoscopy has brought about the greatest change in the technical practice of general surgery in several decades. Together with endoscopic and invasive radiologic techniques for managing surgical disease, laparoscopy represents a clear trend in surgical practice toward the use of minimal-access technology. In just a few years, laparoscopic surgery has revolutionized the management of biliary calculi. During the next decade, similar impacts are likely to be made in other areas of gastrointestinal, oncologic, urologic, and thoracic surgery, and additional applications of laparoscopy are likely to be seen in gynecologic surgery.

This volume examines the current state of laparoscopy in three areas of general surgical practice: herniorrhaphy, intestinal surgery, and biliary tract disease. In each of these areas, current applications of laparoscopy are examined, with emphasis given to data establishing the safety and efficacy of any procedure. A scientifically sound analysis of the current efficacy of laparoscopic techniques is presented. Although the application of laparoscopy in current surgical practice is in a state of constant change, the data and conclusions presented here represent the most recent evidence available through published reports and verbal communications with experts in these areas.

PREFACE

At present, laparoscopic inguinal herniorrhaphy is of great interest to the practicing general surgeon. Because of the large volume of herniorrhaphies performed in surgical practice, the average general surgeon who is accomplished in laparoscopic cholecystectomy but has not used laparoscopy for other procedures is now contemplating the adoption of laparoscopy for herniorrhaphy. It remains to be determined whether laparoscopy will significantly improve postoperative symptoms and recovery of patients undergoing herniorrhaphy as it does of patients undergoing cholecystectomy. The safety and efficacy of laparoscopic herniorrhaphy is being established, and long-term follow-up has been limited.

Laparoscopic intestinal surgery can be categorized as appendiceal and nonappendiceal. Laparoscopic appendectomy was performed years before laparoscopic cholecystectomy; its safety and efficacy have been established in a few centers in Europe. Although its use in general surgical practice in the United States is increasing, there is not sufficient evidence that it represents a clearly improved method of managing appendicitis. However, some patients may especially benefit from laparoscopic appendectomy. These include morbidly obese patients and women of childbearing age who present with lower abdominal pain of uncertain etiology. Laparoscopic intestinal resection (most commonly colon resection) requires laparoscopic surgical skills significantly greater than those required for cholecystectomy. As such, it is likely to be incorporated into surgical practice much more slowly. There are relatively few preliminary data regarding the efficacy of this procedure, although benign intestinal disease appears amenable to laparoscopic resection. Only long-term studies will establish whether laparoscopy can be applied to malignant disease with the same expectation for disease-free survival and cure associated with open procedures.

Laparoscopic cholecystectomy is generally accepted as the treatment of choice for symptomatic cholelithiasis. However,

PREFACE

the problems associated with the safe conduct of this operation are still under examination, and the efficacy of expanding laparoscopic surgical techniques to more complex biliary surgical procedures remains a subject of investigation.

Most of the newer applications of laparoscopy have been made possible by the introduction of special instruments and techniques. Our editors of the first volume of the *Master Series in Surgery* are all leading experts in this field, and each has contributed significantly to the current "state of the art."

Thomas R. Gadacz, MD, has published widely on laparoscopic applications in general surgery. In his section, Dr Gadacz reviews the evolution of laparoscopic methods of hernia repair. He discusses potential complications and expectations of outcome, and offers some cautionary advice for surgeons who are interested in these procedures.

Bruce D. Schirmer, MD, is an expert in laparoscopy, as well as laparoscopic training, and in the pathophysiology of postoperative ileus. In his section, Dr Schirmer discusses laparoscopic bowel resection and laparoscopic appendectomy. He addresses specific indications for laparoscopic techniques, such as coexisting morbid obesity and advanced age, and reviews the current recommendations for laparoscopic enterectomy for benign and malignant disease.

Nathaniel J. Soper, MD, is an expert in the laparoscopic management of biliary disease. In his section, Dr Soper discusses indications, methods, and potential pitfalls in the laparoscopic management of biliary problems. The role of preoperative ERCP and intraoperative cholangiography are reviewed, as well as the role of laparoscopic approaches to acute and complex manifestations of cholecystitis.

Dana K. Andersen, MD

Contributors

Series Editor:

Dana K. Andersen, MD
Professor of Surgery and Medicine
Chief, Section of General Surgery
Department of Surgery
The University of Chicago

Volume Editors:

Thomas R. Gadacz, MD
Professor and Chairman
Department of Surgery
The Medical College of Georgia

Bruce D. Schirmer, MD
Director, Virginia Laparoscopic Institute
Associate Professor of Surgery
University of Virginia

Nathaniel J. Soper, MD
Chief, Gastrointestinal Surgery
Barnes Hospital
Associate Professor of Surgery
Washington University
    School of Medicine

Contents

PREFACE		v
CONTRIBUTORS		viii
Section I	Laparoscopic Hernia Repair	1
	Introduction	1
	Anatomy	2
	Standard Hernia Repair	5
	Laparoscopic Hernia Repair	8
	Indications	8
	Techniques	9
	Results of Inguinal Hernia Repair	13
Section II	Laparoscopic Bowel Resection and Appendectomy	19
	Introduction	19
	Laparoscopic Colon Resection	20
	Method of Segmental Colon Resection	21
	Special Considerations for Rectosigmoid Resection	26
	Results of Laparoscopic Colon Resection	26
	Summary	28

CONTENTS

	Laparoscopic Appendectomy	29
	Indications	29
	Method of Laparoscopic Appendectomy	30
	Results of Laparoscopic Appendectomy	32
	Incidental Appendectomy	33
	Summary	33
	Other Intestinal Surgery	33
Section III	Laparoscopic Treatment of Gallstones	37
	Introduction	38
	Preoperative Considerations	40
	Indications	40
	Contraindications	41
	Equipment	41
	Preoperative Care and Anesthesia	44
	Creation of a Pneumoperitoneum and Trocar Insertion	45
	The Closed Technique	46
	The Open Technique	48
	Technique of Laparoscopic Cholecystectomy	49
	Special Considerations in the Performance of Laparoscopic Cholecystectomy	58
	Anatomic Hazards	58
	Conversion to Open Operation	59
	Acute Cholecystitis	60

Intraoperative Gallbladder Perforation	61
Cholangiography	61
Complications of Laparoscopic Cholecystectomy	62
Postoperative Care	65
Results of Laparoscopic Cholecystectomy	65
Author's Personal Series	65
Other Reported Series	66
Results of the National Institutes of Health Consensus Development Conference	67
Management of Common Bile Duct Stones	68
Conclusion	71
INDEX	74

I Laparoscopic Hernia Repair

Thomas R. Gadacz, MD

BRIEF CONTENTS

Introduction	1
Anatomy	2
Standard Hernia Repair	5
Laparoscopic Hernia Repair	8
Indications	8
Techniques	9
Results of Inguinal Hernia Repair	13

INTRODUCTION

Inguinal hernia repair is one of the oldest operative procedures. Early experience used silk thread for stitching and incorporated all layers of the abdominal wall. A report by Halsted[1] from 1890 described a patient being allowed to get out of bed and walk on the 13th day after herniorrhaphy. Today most inguinal hernia repairs are performed with synthetic sutures, and the patient is ambulatory hours after the operation. Many of the advances in hernia repair have resulted from detailed descriptions of the anatomy and modifications in technique depending upon the type of hernia. The use of prosthetic material to repair hernias originated with the desire to reduce the recurrence of large defects. Laparoscopic hernia repair is an evolving technique, with

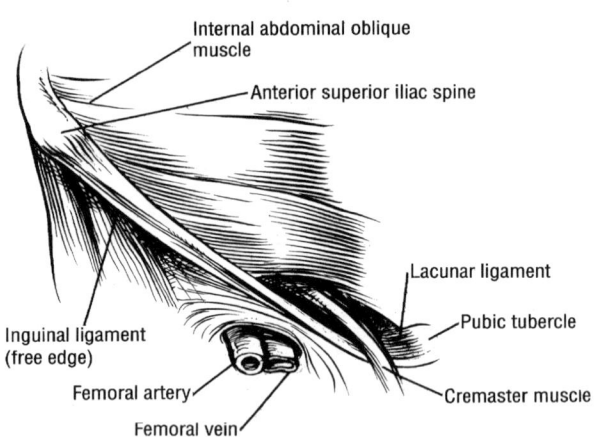

Fig. 1. External view of the inguinal area showing the internal oblique layer and inferior aponeurosis (inguinal ligament) of the external oblique muscle extending from the iliac spine to the pubic tubercle. (Adapted from Knol JA, Eckhauser FE, in Greenfield LJ [ed]. *Surgery: Scientific Principles and Practice*, Philadelphia, Pa, JB Lippincott, 1993, p 1085.)

several types of repairs now being performed. Although many series appear to have favorable outcomes, follow-up has been very short.

ANATOMY

The anatomy of the inguinal area, which has been detailed by Condon[2] and Spaw et al,[3] consists of muscular and tendinous components that permit the protrusion of structures from the abdominal cavity. When structures normally contained in the abdominal cavity protrude through the abdominal wall, a hernia is present. There are three major muscle layers in the inguinal area: the external oblique, the internal oblique, and the transversus abdominis.

Muscles

The external oblique muscle and aponeurosis is the most superficial muscle of the lateral abdominal wall. From attachments on the lower eight ribs, the muscle angles interiorly and medially, inserting on the lateral aponeurosis of the rectus abdominis. The inferior edge forms an aponeurosis from the superior iliac spine to the pubic tubercle and is identified as the inguinal ligament. It folds under itself to form a shelving edge (Fig. 1) and folds 180° at the pubic tubercle to form the lacunar ligament. The internal oblique muscle originates in the area of the iliopsoas. The muscle fibers travel superiorly and obliquely to the lower ribs and are at right angles to the external oblique layer. The cord structures lie beneath the internal oblique layer. The transversus abdominis layer is the deep layer of the lateral abdominal wall. Like

Figure 1

the internal oblique muscle, the transversus muscle originates in the iliopsoas tract but travels transversely and inferiorly. It forms the floor of the inguinal canal and inserts on Cooper's ligament along the superior pubic ramus. The internal oblique and transversus aponeurosis fuse as they insert along the pubic tubercle and superior pubic ramus and form the conjoined tendon. The iliopubic tract belongs to the deep abdominal layer and is part of the transversus aponeurosis extending from the anterior superior iliac spine to the pubic tubercle. It is anterior to the femoral sheath and is associated with the inguinal ligament inferiorly (Fig. 2).

Figure 2
Nerves

The nerve supply to the inguinal area consists of the ilioinguinal and iliohypogastric nerves and the genital branches of the genitofemoral nerves. The ilioinguinal and iliohypogastric nerves arise from the 12th thoracic and first lumbar roots and contain sensory and motor fibers. These two nerves course through the transversus near the iliac crest and the internal oblique near the iliac spine. The ilioinguinal nerve travels on top of the cord and innervates the lateral pubic area and the scrotum or labia. The iliohypogastric nerve lies superior to the internal ring and innervates the suprapubic area. The genital segment of the genitofemoral nerve travels through the transversus inferior to the internal ring and is posterior to the cord. It innervates the lower part of the scrotum and the inner thigh.

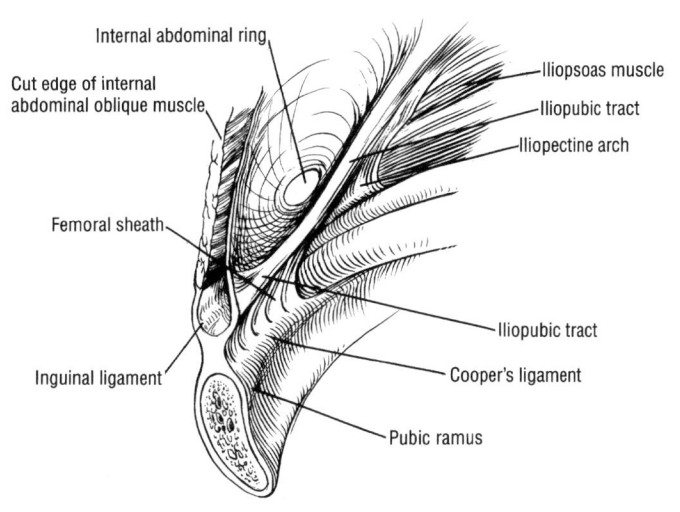

Fig. 2. Internal view of the inguinal area showing the transversus originating from the iliopsoas and forming the iliopubic tract. Superficial to the iliopubic tract is the inguinal ligament, appearing here to cover it. (Adapted from Knol JA, Eckhauser FE, in Greenfield LJ [ed]. *Surgery: Scientific Principles and Practice*, Philadelphia, Pa, JB Lippincott, 1993, p 1086.)

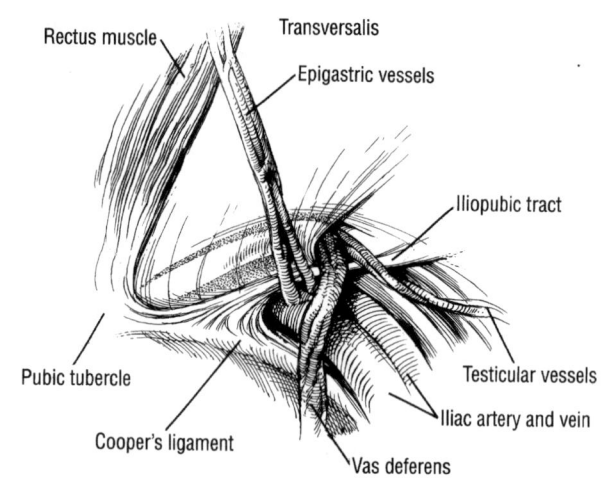

Fig. 3. Schematic view of the right inguinal area through the laparoscope.

Indirect inguinal hernia

There are three types of inguinal hernias that will be considered here: the indirect inguinal hernia, the direct inguinal hernia, and the femoral hernia. The indirect inguinal hernia is the most common type of hernia in children, and is due to a congenital malformation of the shutter mechanism around the internal ring or weakness of the surrounding collagen. In most patients there is a patent processus vaginalis peritonei. The processus vaginalis (testis) is the peritoneal evagination with which the testis descends from the abdomen into the scrotum during the seventh to eighth month in utero. The processus usually obliterates to a fibrous cord, the ligamentum vaginale. The processus may remain open anywhere during its course from the abdomen to the testis. A patent processus provides a potential space for the herniation of intestinal contents into the scrotum. Other potential areas account for hydroceles, and an undescended testicle is almost always associated with an indirect inguinal hernia. In children with an inguinal hernia the internal ring is normal in size; however, in adults the internal ring is usually dilated. The longer the duration of the hernia, the larger the internal ring. An indirect hernia is lateral to the epigastric vessels. Through the laparoscope an indirect hernia is identified as a defect in the peritoneum with the epigastric vessels superior and medial, the vas deferens inferior and medial, and the testicular vessels inferior (Fig. 3).

Direct inguinal hernia

A direct inguinal hernia occurs as the result of a weakness in the transversalis fascia. This area is classically defined as Hesselbach's triangle. It is bounded medially by the lateral border of the rectus abdominis, superiorly by the inferior epigastric vessels, and laterally by the iliopubic tract. Through the laparoscope a direct inguinal hernia appears as a defect medial to the internal ring and epigastric vessels and superior to the iliopubic tract (Fig. 3).

Femoral hernia

A femoral hernia is a defect in the femoral canal and appears as a bulge below the inguinal ligament. The defect is medial to the external iliac vein as it becomes the common femoral vein. In this area the iliopubic tract becomes folded over and attached to Cooper's ligament. Two other fascial boundaries can trap a femoral hernia: the lacunar ligament and the fossa ovalis. Through the laparoscope a femoral hernia appears inferior to the inguinal ligament and medial to the internal ring, ductus deferens, and femoral vessels.

STANDARD HERNIA REPAIR

Hernia repairs can be classified by eponym (eg, Halsted, Bassini, McVay, Shouldice); approach (eg, anterior, posterior, intra-abdominal, laparoscopic); or as nonanatomic or anatomic (Table 1). With the Halsted repair, the floor of the

Table 1

Table 1. Herniorrhaphy: A Glossary

Types of Approach

Anterior: The hernia is approached via the anterior surface of the abdominal wall. This is the most common approach.

Posterior (preperitoneal): The hernia is approached from the posterior aspect of the abdominal wall but anterior to the peritoneum.

Transabdominal: The hernia is approached through the abdomen. The peritoneal lining is penetrated by a laparotomy incision or a laparoscope and cannulas with entrance into the free peritoneal cavity.

Types of Repair

Anatomic: Corresponding layers of the abdominal wall are approximated (eg, the transversus muscle is approximated to the iliopubic tract).

Nonanatomic: Superficial layers of the abdominal wall are approximated to deep layers (eg, the internal oblique muscle is approximated to the iliopubic tract).

Accessories

Sutures: Used to close the hernia defect after the approximation of muscle or aponeurotic layers. Absorbable and nonabsorbable sutures are available.

Staples: Used to close a small defect. They are large and metallic (usually titanium).

Patch: Prosthetic material used to cover the hernia defect. Various types of mesh have been used, including Marlex, Prolene, and polypropylene. Prosthetic material is usually secured with a stapler or sutures.

Plug: A roll of prosthetic material usually inserted into the hernia defect. Its purpose was to obliterate the hernia by inciting an inflammatory reaction. This has been abandoned because of the plug.

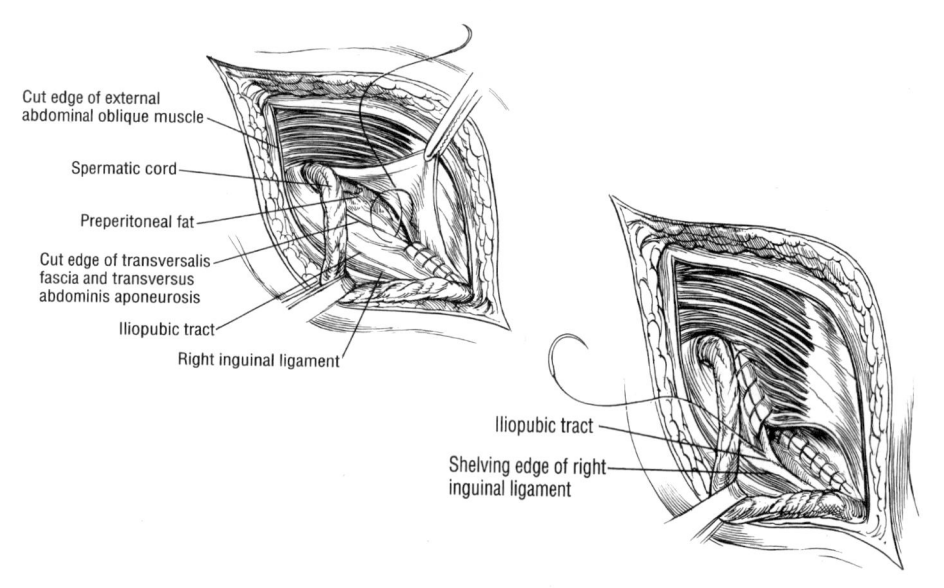

Fig. 4. Anterior view of a Shouldice repair with (A) approximation of the transversus aponeurosis to the transversalis fascia at the lateral border of the rectus, and (B) approximation of the aponeurosis of the transversus and the iliopubic tract. (Adapted from Knol JA, Eckhauser FE, in Greenfield LJ [ed]. *Surgery: Scientific Principles and Practice.* Philadelphia, Pa, JB Lippincott, 1993, p 1096.)

Halsted repair

Bassini repair

McVay repair

Shouldice repair

inguinal canal is reinforced by suturing the transversus muscle (usually including the internal oblique aponeurosis) to the lacunar ligament and the inguinal ligament. This is a nonanatomic repair as it does not approximate muscles in the same layer. This approach is also classified as anterior because the hernia is approached from the skin level (anteriorly). The cord structures are placed in the subcutaneous tissue. The Bassini repair approximates the transversus and internal oblique aponeurosis to the lacunar and inguinal ligaments. This is also considered a nonanatomic repair because more superficial muscles are approximated to deeper structures. As with the Halsted repair, the approach is anterior. The cord structures are placed between the internal and external oblique layers. The McVay repair is used for large direct inguinal and femoral hernias. The transversus is approximated to Cooper's ligament from the pubic tubercle to the femoral canal. Four to 5 cm from the pubic tubercle a transition suture is placed from Cooper's ligament to the transversus abdominis and the anterior femoral sheath. The repair is continued laterally at a more superficial layer approximating the transversus abdominis to the iliopubic tract and the shelving edge of the inguinal ligament. The Shouldice repair[4] involves multiple layers of sutures approximating the

Figure 4

Preperitoneal approach

Figure 5

transversus to transversalis fascia, the iliopubic tract to the shelving edge of the inguinal ligament, and the internal oblique to the inguinal ligament (Fig. 4). Other layers may be approximated.

The posterior or preperitoneal approach was described by Annandale[5] and popularized by Nyhus.[6] The transverse incision is made 3 cm above the pubic tubercle with one third of the incision over the lateral border of the transversus abdominis and two thirds of the incision over the external oblique aponeurosis. The external oblique muscle is spread and the aponeurosis of the internal oblique and transversus muscles are divided lateral to the rectus, exposing the preperitoneal space. The rectus is retracted medially and the fat in the preperitoneal space is dissected off the abdominal wall (Fig. 5).

An indirect hernia is signified by the protrusion of a sack through the internal ring with the cord structures medial to the spermatic cord structures. The sack is dissected away from the cord structures, divided, and ligated. A few sutures are placed in the internal ring to tighten it. A direct hernia is usually a poorly defined sack medial to the inferior epigastric vessels and the internal ring. It appears as a defect in the abdominal wall with the transversus abdominis superior and the iliopubic tract inferior. Cooper's ligament is identified inferiorly and medially and posterior to the pubic tubercle.

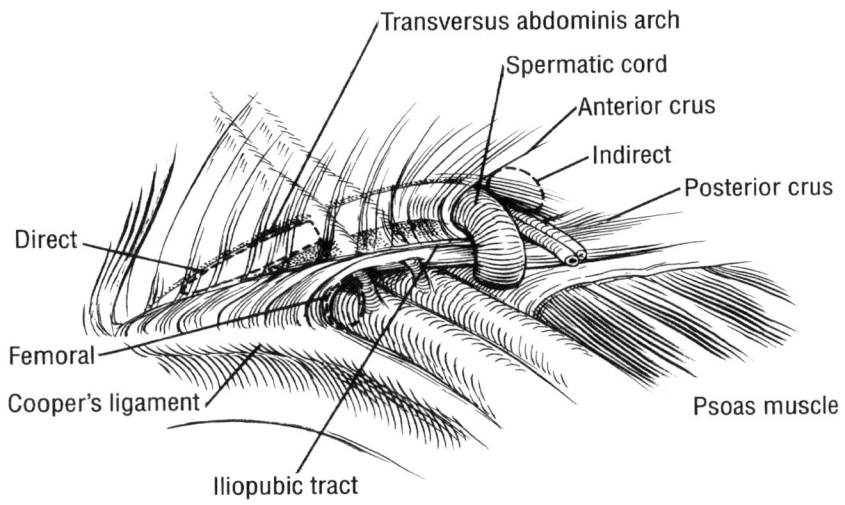

Fig. 5. Schematic view of the inguinal area as visualized by the preperitoneal approach. Locations of indirect, direct, and femoral hernias are indicated. (Adapted from Nyhus LM, in Nyhus LM, Condon RE [eds]. *Hernia*. Philadelphia, Pa, JB Lippincott, 1966, p 218.)

Anatomic repair

The anatomic repair consists of approximating the transversus muscle to the iliopubic tract. If the tissue is attenuated the transversus muscle can be approximated to Cooper's ligament. The transition suture includes the transversus muscle, Cooper's ligament, and the iliopubic tract. The repair is completed by approximating the transversus muscle to the iliopubic tract. A relaxing incision is made along the lateral border of the rectus crossing the transverse incision.

There are several other types of repairs. In 1982 Ger[7] described the intra-abdominal approach to hernia repair, in which the repair was incidental to another major abdominal operation. Today the intra-abdominal approach is used rarely for the primary repair of an inguinal hernia unless there is incarceration and strangulation of the bowel.

The use of prosthetic mesh had become increasingly popular even before the advent of the laparoscopic approach. Mesh was used initially for very large defects but then became popular for a tension-free repair. Lichtenstein[8] used mesh for the repair of direct and indirect inguinal hernias using an anterior approach. He reported good results with no recurrence within 1 to 5 years in 1,000 patients. Stoppa and Warlaumont[9] used mesh in a preperitoneal approach. The advantage to their approach was a low recurrence rate (1.4%) and low incidence of wound problems. These good results were confirmed by Nyhus et al,[10] who reported a recurrence rate of 1.7% in 203 patients.

LAPAROSCOPIC HERNIA REPAIR

In 1990 Popp[11] reported on laparoscopic hernia repair coincidental to a myomectomy. He used dehydrated dura and secured his patch with sutures. In 1991 Schultz[12] reported the use of mesh as a plug and patch, and Corbitt[13] reported the use of a plug and patch with high ligation of the sack. Fitzgibbons[14] has advocated an inlay patch, which consists of a mesh patch covering the defect and held in place with staples. The patch is placed directly on the peritoneum and the hernia sack is not dissected. Others have incised the peritoneum and then covered the mesh with peritoneum after completing the repair. McKernan[15] reported the preperitoneal laparoscopic approach with a patch of mesh. However, this approach is still evolving and the results have not been evaluated adequately.

Indications

Hernias should be repaired to prevent complications of incarceration, strangulation, and bowel obstruction, and to relieve pain. However, the current indications for laparoscopic hernia repair have not been defined. In general, patients with bilateral inguinal hernias and those with a

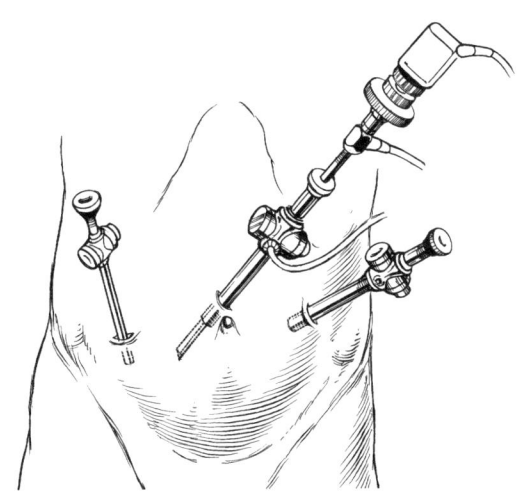

Fig. 6. Schematic view of the position of the cannulas for a laparoscopic right inguinal herniorrhaphy. The cannulas in the umbilical area and left side measure 10 mm and the cannula on the right side measures 5 or 10 mm.

The best candidates for laparoscopic hernia repair

recurrent hernia are the best candidates for laparoscopic herniorrhaphy. The advantages of laparoscopic hernia repair compared with standard Shouldice or Lichtenstein repair have not been established, but clinical observations suggest that patients undergoing laparoscopic herniorrhaphy require less pain medication, ambulate earlier with less restricted motion, and have a shorter recovery time.

Techniques

Three techniques of inguinal hernia repair will be discussed here. Two methods involve a transperitoneal approach and one method involves a preperitoneal approach. The trans-

Two methods of transperitoneal repair

peritoneal technique consists of establishing a pneumoperitoneum in a standard fashion with carbon dioxide. Cannulas are inserted using a trocar. A 10-mm cannula in the umbilical area is used for the laparoscope, and a 5- or 10-mm port is inserted in the midabdominal area at the lateral border of the rectus and the level of the umbilicus on the side of the hernia. The dissection and retraction are performed through this cannula. A 10- to 12-mm cannula is then inserted in the midabdominal area on the contralateral side, also at the border of the rectus and the level of the umbilicus. The hernia is dissected through this port, and the stapler is inserted to

Figure 6

secure a prosthesis. Figure 6 shows the position of the cannulas for a right inguinal hernia repair. Following a general inspection of the abdominal cavity, the inguinal area is inspected. The patient is placed in a Trendelenburg position with the monitor at the foot of the operating table. The groin and scrotum should be prepped, as manipulation of the hernia may assist identification and repair of the defect. The epigastric and iliac vessels must be identified to prevent injury; the vas deferens and testicular vessels should be identified, as well. Figure 3 illustrates the relationship of these structures. Subsequent steps in the operation depend upon the chosen technique but many of the steps are similar. Identification of the anatomy is the most important part of the operation. Using the inlay technique of Fitzgibbons,[14] the hernia sack is not dissected but the contents of the hernia are reduced. Mesh is positioned over the hernia defect and stapled into place. Fitzgibbons favors polypropylene mesh. Limited clinical experience is available for this approach.

Another approach involves the transperitoneal technique but the peritoneum over the hernia is incised and the mesh is placed on the posterior aspect of the abdominal wall. Initially the procedure consisted of inserting a plug of polypropylene in the hernia defect and covering the defect with a polypropylene patch. The patch was covered by approximating the peritoneum over the mesh. However, this technique was soon modified to stapling the mesh in place to prevent migration and herniation. The purpose of the plug was to incite an inflammatory response to obliterate the defect with scarring. The problem with this technique was the migration of the plugs and patch into the groin and scrotum; the technique was abandoned quickly because of poor outcome even when the plug was sutured to the patch to prevent migration. Small patches were used initially, but these tended to herniate into the inguinal canal, or a hernia would occur around an edge of the patch. The use of larger patches followed, and some of the techniques of Lichtenstein and Stoppa were applied to laparoscopic hernia repair. As the procedure was modified and staples were used routinely to secure the mesh in place, the size of the mesh increased gradually, and large flaps of peritoneum were developed to cover the mesh. In current practice the mesh extends from the pubic tubercle medially to a ridge along Cooper's ligament, continuing laterally along the iliopubic tract, superiorly along the transversalis fascia, and laterally beyond the internal ring. The lateral part of the mesh is usually incised so that the internal ring and cord structures can be covered. Figure 7 shows the mesh in place.

Figure 7

Once the hernia is identified, the area between the vas deferens and the spermatic vessels is noted and avoided. In this area (sometimes referred to as the triangle of doom) lie the iliac vessels. The peritoneum is incised, beginning medial to the vas deferens, to expose Cooper's ligament and the iliopubic tract. The peritoneum is dissected carefully off the

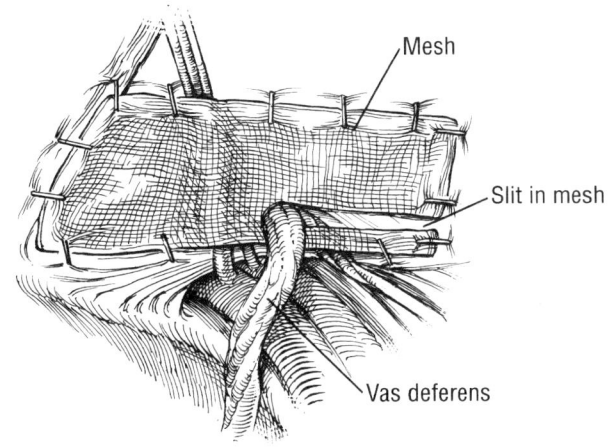

Fig. 7. Prosthetic material stapled to the inguinal area in a transperitoneal laparoscopic herniorrhaphy.

inferior epigastric vessels. An indirect hernia is reduced and the neck is ligated just below the internal ring (high ligation). The ring can be tightened with a few sutures or the entire floor reinforced with a 5 × 10-cm piece of mesh. The mesh is rolled and passed into the abdomen through the larger cannula and unrolled against the hernia defect. A grasper in the ipsilateral cannula holds the mesh in place; a stapler is passed through the contralateral cannula to secure the mesh. Several sutures are placed in Cooper's ligament beginning at the pubic tubercle lateral to the iliopubic tract. The mesh is secured superiorly along the transversus muscle, beginning at the pubic tubercle and ending lateral to the internal ring. Although some staples are placed lateral to the internal ring, staples along the lateral border should be avoided to prevent injury to the genital branch of the genitofemoral nerve. The area is usually irrigated and the irrigant is aspirated. The pneumoperitoneum is reduced to a pressure of 5 to 6 mm Hg and the peritoneum is approximated over the mesh with staples or titanium clips. The surrounding area is inspected for hemostasis, the pneumoperitoneum is released, and the cannulas are removed.

The same exposure is necessary for repair of a direct inguinal hernia. This hernia is located between the epigastric vessels and the lateral border of the rectus abdominis. It is not necessary to excise the hernia sack but the prosthesis needs to cover the entire area, as described previously.

Preperitoneal method

The preperitoneal approach, described by McKernan,[15]

Table 2. Series of Hernia Repairs

Type of Repair	Reference	Patients (n)	Recurrence (%)	Follow-Up
General	16	—(survey)	10.0	Years
Lichtenstein	8	1,000	0.0	1-5 yr
Nyhus	10	203	1.7	Years
TA*	12	20	0.0	<1 yr
TA	20	10	0.0	6 mo
TA	18	36	0.0	1 yr
PP**	15	25	0.0	1 yr

*TA = Laparoscopic transperitoneal approach. Some of these procedures are termed preperitoneal by the authors; however, this refers to the position of the prosthesis.

**PP = Laparoscopic preperitoneal approach. This refers to the procedure being performed in the preperitoneal space with the peritoneum in the inguinal area not being incised (except to transect the neck of the sack of an indirect hernia).

begins with a midline umbilical incision. The fascia is incised and the preperitoneal space is entered but not violated. A preperitoneal space is developed with the laparoscope; instillation of saline or insufflation with carbon dioxide exposes the inguinal area. Two lateral cannulas are inserted, and the dissection is similar to that with the transperitoneal approach. Identification of the internal ring and hernia is important because the orientation is different. The preperitoneal fat must be pushed inferiorly to expose the posterior aspect of the abdominal wall. The inferior epigastric vessels, Cooper's ligament, femoral vessels, and ductus deferens are identified next and the hernia is repaired. An indirect hernia can be reduced if it is small; if it is extensive, the sack can be transected and ligated. Direct hernias are reduced. Placement of the prosthesis is similar to that described for the transperitoneal approach. McKernan cuts a slit in the prosthesis to fit around the cord, and uses a 4.5 x 7.5-cm patch of polypropylene.

There are some modifications to the preperitoneal approach, including the use of a transperitoneal (intra-abdominal) cannula and laparoscope to guide the placement of a Veress needle in the preperitoneal space. This way the space can be developed by carbon dioxide insufflation. Once the preperitoneal space is developed, three cannulas are introduced and hernia repair is performed.

We have used an inflatable retractor attached to a cannula to develop the preperitoneal space. This technique has the advantage of dissecting the area without forcing carbon dioxide or saline into the surrounding tissues. The direction of the retractor can be controlled by the cannula, and the surrounding tissues are compressed. This optimizes exposure of the area. Following withdrawal of the inflatable retractor, carbon dioxide insufflation will depress the peritoneum and provide a good operative field.

The best approach has yet to emerge

The techniques thus described indicate that the best laparoscopic approach has not yet emerged. The clinical trials evaluating these techniques are incomplete. The most important outcome is recurrence rate. Complications from the prostheses are not fully known, but the experience with prosthetic material for standard hernia repair does not suggest the likelihood of a high complication rate. Preliminary studies we performed on pigs in our laboratory indicate a higher rate of adhesions to the hernia site when the transperitoneal approach is used than when the preperitoneal approach is used. The clinical significance of this observation is not known, but it does suggest that the preperitoneal approach may be the technique of choice.

RESULTS OF INGUINAL HERNIA REPAIR

The results of laparoscopic inguinal hernia repair are known in a limited number of cases with very short follow-ups. The procedure is still undergoing technical modifications. Table 2 lists the results from some series using conventional repairs and others involving laparoscopic herniorrhaphy.

Table 2

Table 3

Table 3 details some of the reports on laparoscopic herniorrhaphy. MacFayden[16] reported on 359 laparoscopic

Table 3. Summary of Results of Laparoscopic Hernia Repair

	Number of Hernias (% Failures)		
Series	Direct	Indirect	Follow-Up (Months)
Arregui*	37 (0%)	57 (0%)	28
Bogojavalensky[22]	9 (11%)	30 (3%)	41
Corbitt[13]	12 (8%)	23 (9%)	15
Filipi[23]	49 (2%)	31 (3%)	13
Ger*	3 (0%)	24 (4%)	64
Phillips[24]	39 (0%)	23 (0%)	10

*Unpublished

herniorrhaphies performed in several centers, with a follow-up of 13 to 104 months. The recurrence rate was 0.8%, and the incidence of complications was 10%. These complications included hematomas of the scrotum, inguinal canal, and anterior abdominal wall; bladder injury; hydrocele of the scrotum; and pain in the cord and anterior thigh. One patient developed osteitis pubis.

Method according to Gazayerli

Gazayerli[17] reported on 14 patients who underwent laparoscopic repair of inguinal hernias (four indirect, nine direct, and one recurrent). He described a technique in which four cannulas were employed: A 10-mm cannula is inserted in the umbilical area for the laparoscope, a 12-mm cannula is inserted at McBurney's point on the contralateral side, a second 10-mm cannula is inserted at the level of the umbilicus and at the lateral border of the rectus on the side of the hernia, and a 10-mm cannula is inserted between the pubic tubercle and epigastric vessels cephalad to the hernia. Through the cannula near the hernia a specialized abdominal wall retractor is inserted for exposure. The hernia is then repaired with a combination of suturing and mesh techniques. The posterior wall is approximated with two or three sutures through the transversalis and iliopubic tract, and a roll of Marlex mesh is placed in the defect and additional sutures are positioned to close the defect. In two patients a relaxing incision was made in the transversalis muscle and a piece of polypropylene mesh was sutured over the relaxing incision. In two patients the laparoscopic approach was converted to an open procedure. In one of these patients there were problems maintaining a pneumoperitoneum and in the other there were problems with exposure because of a prior operation. The initial case required 211 minutes; the current range is between 90 and 180 minutes. All patients were discharged within 23 hours following the operation, and no complications were reported.

Corbitt's series

Corbitt[13] reported on 20 patients (18 men and two women) undergoing laparoscopic herniorrhaphy with a plug and patch technique. Thirteen patients had indirect hernias and seven patients had direct hernias. The longest follow-up in this series was 8 months, and no complications were reported.

Method of Arregui et al

Arregui et al[18] reported on 52 patients (50 men and two women) who underwent 61 laparoscopic preperitoneal hernia repairs. Thirty-eight hernias were indirect, 22 hernias were direct, and one hernia was femoral. Twenty-five patients had a hernia on the right side, 19 patients had a hernia on the left side, and eight patients had bilateral hernias. Twelve hernias were recurrent, with an equal distribution between sides. The procedure involved a transabdominal approach with repair of the posterior abdominal wall and approximation of the peritoneum over the mesh. In this technique, a 5 x 11.5-cm nonabsorbable mesh is placed over the internal ring, Cooper's ligament, pubic symphysis, and transversus muscle. The mesh is secured with three 3-0 Vicryl sutures. The sutures are then placed superiorly in the transversalis fascia and transversus aponeurosis, inferiorly in Cooper's ligament or the iliopubic tract, and laterally in the transversus lateral to the internal ring. The peritoneum is closed with a continuous 3-0 Vicryl suture. No intraoperative complications occurred but three postoperative complications (5.8%) were reported. Two patients had hematomas of the scrotum, and one patient had right testicular swelling that lasted for 7 days. Duration of follow-up was 2.3 months, during which time there were no recurrences.

Procedure according to Seid et al

Seid et al[19] reported on 27 patients who underwent 29 laparoscopic hernia repairs. Eighteen hernias were indirect, nine hernias were direct, and two hernias were femoral. Four patients had bilateral hernias, which were repaired simultaneously. Employing a transabdominal approach, with a roll of polypropylene plugs attached to a 4 x 4-cm sheet, two 4 x 6-cm patches are placed over the defect. One of the larger patches is placed medial to the epigastric vessels and the other is attached lateral to the epigastric vessels, over the internal ring. All procedures were performed on an outpatient basis, and the only complication reported was postoperative urinary retention, which occurred in one patient. Duration of follow-up was 1 to 7 months, with no recurrence reported in 25 of the 27 patients. Full employment was achieved in 3 to 7 days.

Technique of Toy and Smoot

Toy and Smoot[20] reported on ten patients (seven men and three women) who underwent 11 laparoscopic hernia repairs. Nine hernias were indirect and two hernias were direct. One patient had bilateral indirect hernias. With the transabdominal approach the authors employed, the operating cannula is inserted into the umbilical area and two lateral cannulas are inserted into the anterior axillary line at the level of the umbilicus. A 5 x 7-cm piece of polytetrafluoroethylene with a thickness of 1 mm is used to cover the defect. The peritoneum is not incised, but an indirect sack is ligated or transected, similar to the inlay technique of Fitzgibbons.[14] The procedure lasted from 70 to 129 minutes, with a mean of 90.8 minutes. Bilateral hernia repair took the longest time. There were no complications. Duration of follow-up was 3 to 6 months, and no recurrences were reported.

Method of McKernan and Laws

Finally, McKernan and Laws[21] reported on 25 patients who underwent preperitoneal laparoscopic hernia repair. In this procedure a preperitoneal space is developed by dissecting through a 2-cm umbilical incision. The space is insufflated with carbon dioxide at a pressure of 8 to 10 mm Hg. Two cannulas are then placed in the midline: a 12-mm cannula

Table 4. Potential Complications of Laparoscopic Herniorrhaphy

Complications related to laparoscopy

    Gas embolism
    Trocar injury (vessel, bladder, bowel)
    Cautery injury (bowel, bladder)

Complications related to laparoscopic hernia repair

    Vascular injury
    Bladder/bowel injury
    Injury to the vas deferens
    Migration of the prosthesis
    Infection of the prosthesis
    Adhesions with bowel obstruction
    Nerve injury
    Recurrence of the hernia

midway between the umbilicus and the pubic symphysis, and a 5-mm cannula 1 cm above the pubis. A 7.5 x 12.5-cm mesh is placed over the inguinal area. Next, a 1.5-in slit is cut 2 in from the cephalad portion in the mesh. The cord structures pass through the lower part of this slit. The testicular vessels and the ductus deferens are dissected away from the posterior abdominal wall and the mesh passes behind these structures. Although the patients in this series have not been followed, no intraoperative complications have been reported. However, one patient (4.2%) developed subcutaneous fluid collection following repair of an indirect hernia and two patients (8.3%) developed subcutaneous fluid collections following repair of a large direct hernia. In two patients the fluid was reabsorbed within 1 week; in the third patient, aspiration was required at 2 weeks, with no reaccumulation of the fluid.

Apparently few complications

Reports on complications of laparoscopic herniorrhaphy seem to follow a pattern similar to that of initial reports with laparoscopic cholecystectomy. In almost all of the reported series no complications have occurred, yet there are anecdotal reports of injuries to the vessels (usually inferior epigastric) and ductus deferens. Although there are references to the triangle of doom (the area between the vas deferens and the testicular vessels wherein lie the iliac vessels), there have been no reports of severe bleeding from iliac vessel injury.

Table 4

More than likely, however, injuries have occurred (Table 4).

References
1. Halsted WS. *Bull Johns Hopkins Hosp* 1890;1:111-112.
2. Condon RE, in Nyhus LM, Condon RE (eds). *Hernia*, Philadelphia, Pa, JB Lippincott, 1989, pp 18-64.
3. Spaw AT, et al. *J Laparosc Surg* 1991;1:269-277.
4. Shearburn EW, Myers RN. *Surgery* 1969;66:540-549.
5. Annandale T. *Edinburgh Med J* 1876;21:1087.
6. Nyhus LM, et al. *West J Surg* 1959;67:48.
7. Ger R. *Ann R Coll Surg Engl* 1982;64:342-344.
8. Lichtenstein IL, et al. *Am J Surg* 1989;157:188-193.
9. Stoppa RE, Warlaumont CR, in Nyhus LM, Condon RE (eds). *Hernia*, Philadelphia, Pa, JB Lippincott, 1989, pp 199-225.
10. Nyhus LM, et al. *Ann Surg* 1988;208:733-737.
11. Popp LW. *Surg Endosc* 1990;4:10-12.
12. Schultz L, et al. *J Laparoendosc Surg* 1990;1:41-45.
13. Corbitt JD Jr. *Surg Laparosc Endosc* 1991;1:23-25.
14. Salerno GM, et al, in Zucker KA (ed). *Surgical Laparoscopy*, St Louis, Mo, Quality Medical Publishing 1991, pp 281-293.
15. McKernan JB. *Laparoscopic Focus* 1992;1:1-12.
16. MacFayden B. *SAGES Symposium* 1992;5:9-10.
17. Gazayerli MM. *Surg Laparosc Endosc* 1992;2:49-52.
18. Arregui ME, et al. *Surg Laparosc Endosc* 1992;2:53-58.
19. Seid AS, et al. *Surg Laparosc Endosc* 1992;2:59-60.
20. Toy FK, Smoot RT. *Surg Laparosc Endosc* 1991;1:151-155.
21. McKernan JE, Laws HL. *Surg Rounds* 1992; :597-610.
22. Bogojavalensky S. *Laparoscopic Treatment of Inguinal and Femoral Hernia* (videotape). Presented at the 15th Annual Meeting of the American Association of Gynecologic Laparoscopists, Washington, DC, 1989.
23. Filipi CJ, et al. *Surg Clin North Am* 1992;72:1109-1123.
24. Phillips EH. *Laparoscopic Focus* 1992;1:1-12.

II Laparoscopic Bowel Resection and Appendectomy

Bruce D. Schirmer, MD

BRIEF CONTENTS

Introduction	19
Laparoscopic Colon Resection	20
Method of Segmental Colon Resection	21
Special Considerations for Rectosigmoid Resection	26
Results of Laparoscopic Colon Resection	26
Summary	28
Laparoscopic Appendectomy	29
Indications	29
Method of Laparoscopic Appendectomy	30
Results of Laparoscopic Appendectomy	32
Incidental Appendectomy	33
Summary	33
Other Intestinal Surgery	33

INTRODUCTION

Laparoscopic intestinal surgery is currently in its early stages. Although laparoscopic appendectomy has been practiced in several European clinics for many years, it had achieved only limited popularity until recently. Colon surgery, particularly resection, is the most widely performed intestinal surgery. Therefore, this discussion will focus on colon resection and appendectomy as representative of the current state of laparoscopic intestinal surgery. Small bowel resection, gastrojejunostomy, placement of laparoscopic jejunostomy tubes, and numerous other intestinal procedures have been performed using laparoscopic techniques. However, the two procedures that form the basis of this discussion involve most of the skills needed and principles that underlie these other procedures and are, based on their current popularity, worthy of special attention.

LAPAROSCOPIC COLON RESECTION

Demanding advanced laparoscopic skills

Laparoscopic colon resection is a formidable undertaking for the surgeon. It requires advanced laparoscopic skills including facility with two-handed dissection, extracorporeal knot-tying, intracorporeal knot-tying and suturing, and the ability to retract organs via the laparoscope without causing iatrogenic injury. It is recommended that the surgeon spend considerable time and effort preparing for the performance of such a procedure. The necessary skills should be developed in an inanimate suturing laboratory and by performing the procedure itself on a live animal model.

"Laparoscopic-assisted colon resection" may be a more accurate term

The term laparoscopic colon resection may be misleading, as most surgeons still perform the anastomosis extracorporeally. This is practical, time-sparing, and effective because an incision of adequate size is needed to remove the resected specimen and complete the procedure. It also may be possible to complete division of a portion of the mesentery extracorporeally, but this should not be included in the preoperative plan as it is impossible to predict whether full mobilization of the segment of colon to be resected will allow removal through the abdominal wall without prior intracorporeal mesenteric division. Thus, the term laparoscopic-assisted colon resection is probably more accurate to describe the procedure most commonly performed. The only exception would be low anterior resection or segmental sigmoid resection, where the specimen is removed transanally by means of a colonoscope. In such a situation, standard trocar-size wounds may suffice to complete the procedure. Yet even here the popular use of the circular stapling device necessitates that at least one of these wounds be large enough to accommodate the circular anvil of the stapler. Thus, in this discussion the term laparoscopic colon resection will be used to describe all colon resections involving the laparoscopic approach.

Table 1

Current indications for laparoscopic colon resection are listed in Table 1. The benign conditions are all relative indications, assuming sufficient evidence that the safety and

Table 1. Indications for Performing Laparoscopic Colon Resection

Benign Conditions	
Colonic polyposis	Volvulus
Villous polyps	Stricture
AV malformations (as a cause of bleeding)	Rectal prolapse
	Inflammatory bowel disease
Diverticular disease	Trauma
Colonic inertia	Ischemic colitis

Malignant Conditions
Palliative resection
Duke's A lesions (polyps)
Curative resection

Resection for neoplasm is still controversial

efficacy of such an approach are not in question. Much more controversial are the neoplastic conditions for which the procedure is currently being performed. It will take several years of follow-up to determine whether patients undergoing laparoscopic colon resection for adenocarcinoma of the colon have experienced a compromise of their treatment. Advocates of extending the procedure to neoplastic indications have cited the fact that the number of lymph nodes harvested in the surgical specimens is not significantly different from the number obtained during open colon resection. In addition, once experience with segmental dissection is attained, it may be possible to replicate the resection as it would be performed in an open manner. We have found this to be true for right hemicolectomy and segmental sigmoid resection.

Method of Segmental Colon Resection

The patient is prepared in the usual manner, with a thorough mechanical and antibiotic bowel preparation to lessen the risk of perioperative infection. Parenteral antibiotics may be administered at the time of surgery, although there is insufficient evidence that they provide additional benefit given adequate bowel preparation. The patient must be counseled about the procedure, with information given regarding the surgeon's experience with laparoscopic colon resection, the potential for conversion to open laparotomy, and the experimental nature of the laparoscopic colon resection, especially when used to treat carcinoma.

The operating team

The operating team consists of a surgeon, a first assistant, a camera operator, and a scrub nurse. Personnel can be arranged according to the surgeon's preference, but we have found that the optimal arrangement is to place the surgeon on the side opposite the section of colon to be resected. The camera operator should stand close to the surgeon, and the assistant should stand on either side of the table or between the patient's legs in order to optimally assist. The lithotomy position is indicated when a mucosal lesion is to be removed and intraoperative localization of the lesion may be necessary. In such situations, we have found that intraoperative colonoscopy performed by a member of the surgical team is highly effective (hence, the need for the lithotomy position for access to the anus). However, if the colonoscopist can inject india ink into the submucosa of the colon at the site of the lesion preoperatively, such a procedure may be avoided. Of course, it is never a certainty that the india ink will be clearly visible upon laparoscopic inspection of the colon. The lithotomy position is also indicated for left-sided colon or rectal resection, as it allows the option of a transrectal stapled anastomosis.

Trocar port positioning is variable, based on the location of the bowel segment to be removed (Fig. 1). General principles for port placement include (1) accommodating the telescope as far across the abdomen as possible, allowing the widest view of the operative field; (2) placing the ports according to the laparoscopic visualization of the anatomy, as the proce-

Figure 1

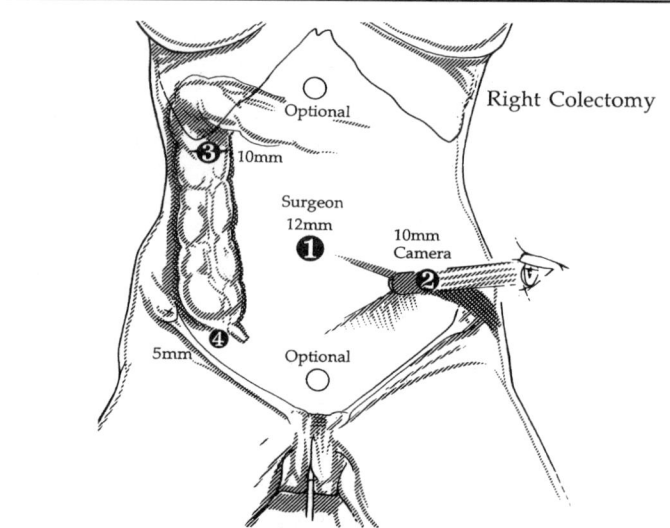

Fig. 1. Recommended port placement for laparoscopic right colon resection. Port no. 1 is used for one of the surgeon's hands. The optional site in either the epigastric or suprapubic region (depending on the location of the segment of colon to be resected) is used for the surgeon's other hand. Placement of port no. 2 in the left abdominal area allows a wider range of view for the telescope. Ports nos. 3 and 4 are used for retraction and exposure early in the procedure. Port no. 4 is situated where the intestinal anastomosis is anticipated, allowing placement of a larger port (such as a 10-mm port) in this location.

Table 2. Steps Involved in Laparoscopic Colon Resection

---

1. Mobilization by incising lateral peritoneal reflection
2. Incision of peritoneal mesentery medially
3. Clear identification of ureter if in the area of dissection
4. Definition of the location of the lesion to be resected
5. Determination of limits of bowel resection
6. Suspension of bowel to expose mesentery to be divided
7. Division of mesentery to involved segment*
8. Division of bowel proximally and distally*
9. Removal of specimen
10. Creation of bowel anastomosis*
11. Replacement of bowel into peritoneal cavity
12. Closure of any mesenteric defect

*Optionally performed extracorporeally in part or in total.

---

dure progresses; (3) placing a large port in a location likely to be used later for a small open incision for retrieving the specimen and performing extracorporeal anastomosis; (4) placing the ports relatively far apart, to prevent interference ("sword fighting") with one another during the procedure; (5) placing ports to avoid the line of vision of the telescope; and (6) placing the ports far enough from each side of the telescope port to allow the surgeon to work comfortably in a two-handed manner.

The size of the ports to be placed varies with the surgeon's preference and the instruments required from that position. Some laparoscopic surgeons have advocated the use of all 10- to 12-mm ports to allow optimal instrumental flexibility with each port. Currently a 12-mm port is required for a short (30-mm) anastomotic stapling device, and a port measuring ≥15 mm is required for a larger (60-mm) stapling device.

Table 2, Figure 2

The steps involved in laparoscopic colon resection are summarized in Table 2 and illustrated in Fig. 2. Lateral peritoneal mobilization is facilitated by table positioning to optimally expose the lateral abdominal side wall to be dissected. We have found the disposable scissors equipped with electrocautery to be most effective for performing this dissection. Larger vessels in the area of the hepatic or splenic flexure should be ligated or clipped to achieve complete hemostasis, as cautery is often insufficient. Every effort should be made to keep bleeding to a minimum during this portion of the operation, as this will aid in identification of the ureter. Mobilization of the right and left colon is

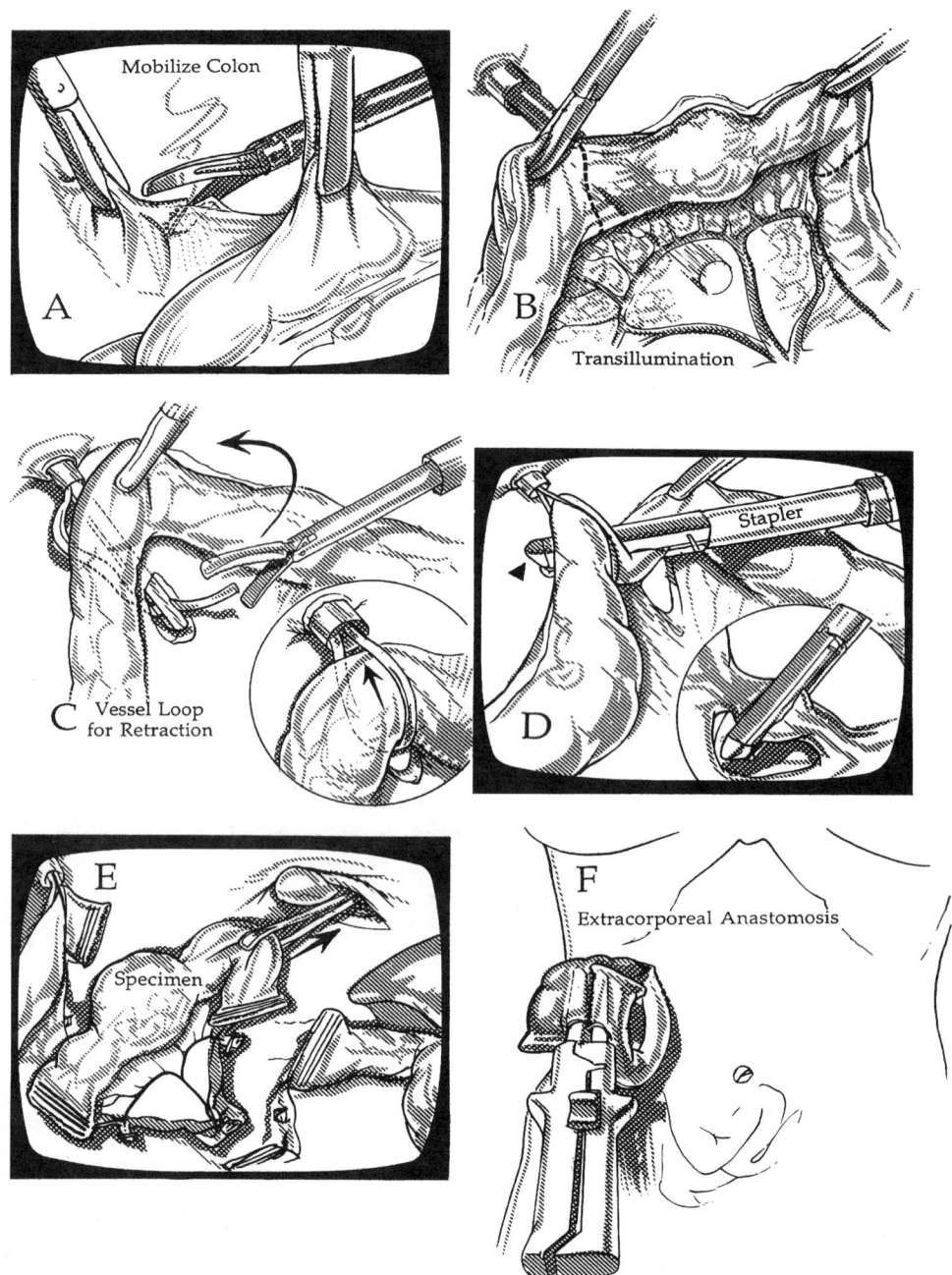

Fig. 2. Sequence of steps in right colon resection. (A) Mobilization of the colon by incision of the lateral peritoneal attachments. (B) Transillumination, by a second light source and telescope, of the mesentery to define the locations of bowel and mesenteric division following location of the lesion to be removed. (C) Placement of vessel loops for retraction of the colon at the points of proposed bowel division. (D) Use of the endoscopic stapler to divide the bowel and a major vascular pedicle. (E) Extraction of the resected segment of colon through a small incision made at the location of port no. 3. Placement in a protective bag (not shown) can be used if needed to prevent wound contamination. (F) Extracorporeal anastomosis using a GIA-type stapler performed between the two ends of bowel that also have been brought out through the small wound.

technically easier than mobilization of the transverse colon. The latter presents the problem of removing the omentum from the colon. Laparoscopic exposure of the hepatic flexure is also less difficult than exposure of the splenic flexure.

Localization of the lesion and suspension of the colon

Identification of the lesion to be resected is often obvious under laparoscopic inspection of the colon. When it is not, intraoperative colonoscopy is performed to localize the lesion. The extent of resection is then determined, and the bowel is suspended at the points of future intestinal resection. We have found vessel loops useful for accomplishing this. The vessel loop is passed around the bowel adjacent to its serosal surface. The two ends of the loop are then brought out through a port and clamped together. The port can still be used to accommodate an instrument. Suspension of the bowel in this manner allows the mesentery to be exposed optimally, like a curtain, permitting good visualization of the major mesenteric vessels.

Division of the mesentery can be accomplished safely in a variety of ways. If the mesentery is thick or fatty, transillumination using a second light source and a 5-mm telescope is often helpful. The major vessels must be identified clearly in order to be ligated safely. The relatively avascular areas of the mesentery can be divided with the electrocautery scissors. Vessels can be secured with ligatures, the vascular stapler, or clips. We prefer to divide and

Dividing the mesentery and securing the major vessels

secure the major vessels using one of the former two methods, reserving clips for smaller vessels or vessel lumens of the specimen side of a divided vessel. Passing long ($\geq$36-in) ligatures around an isolated vascular arcade and using extracorporeally tied knots allows a relatively rapid and secure ligation of the vessels. Although the vascular stapler is more rapid, it is less cost-effective. However, the vascular stapler (with a more proximal Roeder loop ligature) is an extremely reliable way of securing the major vessels.

If the bowel is divided intracorporeally, a stapling device should be used. This avoids the potential of intraperitoneal spillage of bowel contents. The recent availability of endoscopic GIA- and TA-type staplers in 60-mm lengths allows intracorporeal intestinal anastomosis with a total stapling technique. Compared with hand-sewing an anastomosis intracorporeally, stapling lessens operating time, a significant advantage. In addition, stapling devices allow the creation of an anastomosis when full mobilization of the resected ends of the bowel does not allow them to reach comfortably outside the peritoneal cavity. However, when bowel mobilization easily allows the ends to be brought outside the peritoneal cavity, there is no advantage to intracorporeal anastomosis over extracorporeal anastomosis.

Intracorporeal vs extracorporeal stapling

In removing a resected specimen of bowel, care must be

taken to avoid wound contamination and potential tumor seeding. To this end, it is helpful to introduce a plastic bag into the peritoneal cavity for placement of the specimen.

Special Considerations for Rectosigmoid Resection

The initial approach to rectosigmoid resection is similar to that to other segmental colon resections. (Figure 3 illustrates the sigmoid colectomy procedure.) Incision of the mesenteric peritoneum on both sides of the rectosigmoid should allow the clear identification of both ureters. Division of the vascular blood supply to the area involves the proximal division of the superior hemorrhoidal artery or inferior mesenteric artery, based on the lesion and its malignant potential. Steep Trendelenburg position and a broad bowel retractor are often necessary to allow adequate exposure of these vessels in their retroperitoneal location beneath the overlying loops of small intestine.

Division of the middle hemorrhoidal vessels is performed using any of the aforementioned techniques for secure vascular division. Clips are not favored as they can be dislodged easily during further dissection and manipulation. Adequate pelvic exposure, which may be difficult to achieve, requires the placement of ports near the suprapubic area to allow instruments to reach deep into the pelvis.

Distal rectosigmoid bowel division is usually best accomplished with a stapling device. In some instances, a suprapubic incision is necessary to accommodate an extracorporeal device, the roticulating head of which has not been replicated in an endoscopic stapler to date. When a suprapubic incision is made, mobilization of the proximal end of resected bowel through the wound in an extracorporeal location allows the anvil portion of a circular stapling device to be secured into the bowel lumen by a purse-string suture. The shaft of the stapling device is then introduced transanally, and a circular stapled anastomosis is performed via a standard technique. Security of the anastomosis is tested routinely using air or colored liquid (eg, methylene blue in saline) introduced through the rectum.

Results of Laparoscopic Colon Resection

There are few published results of laparoscopic colon resection. However, the results that are available in published and preliminary form, including our own experience with over 20 cases of laparoscopic colon surgery, illustrate several main points: (1) Laparoscopic colon surgery is feasible and may be performed safely for many indications; (2) most surgeons have initiated their experience with this procedure for nonmalignant conditions of the colon; (3) most surgeons have used a laparoscopic-assisted technique, making a small incision to perform an extracorporeal anastomosis; (4) morbidity and mortality have been acceptably low in most cases; (5) hospital stay and time to recovery may be shorter than that required for open colon operations; and (6) certain operations (eg, right segmental colectomy, sigmoid colectomy) may be performed laparoscopically with equal therapeutic effect for malignant lesions. This assumption is based on the fact that similar numbers of lymph nodes are included in the specimens of laparoscopic colectomies and open colectomies. However, long-term follow-up will be needed before this hypothesis can be confirmed.

Experience at other centers

Jacobs et al[1] have reported on a series of 20 patients undergoing laparoscopic-assisted colectomies (overwhelmingly right or sigmoid colectomies). Eighty percent of patients were able to tolerate a liquid diet on the first postoperative day and 70% of patients were discharged within 4 days. Fifteen percent of patients experienced operative complications. Other cases of successful laparoscopic colon resection have been reported with similar rapid postoperative recovery.[2,3] However, Wexner et al[4] reported no improvement in recovery from postoperative ileus or decrease in hospital stay among a group of patients who had undergone total abdominal colectomy using the laparoscopic approach. Operative time was 35% longer for the patients who had undergone laparoscopy than those who had undergone standard laparotomy.

Unpublished larger series of colectomies have been reported in course syllabus form.[5] For the most part these preliminary data further confirm the efficacy of laparoscopic colectomy, although in one series the conversion rate to celiotomy was 41%. Hospital stay was longer for patients undergoing initial celiotomy or conversion to celiotomy. One surgeon's experience showed that operating time for laparoscopic sigmoid colectomy decreased by 50% over a 10-month period. This suggests a significant learning curve that implies a shorter duration of surgery with increasing experience. This may have a significant impact on the cost-effectiveness of laparoscopic colectomy in the future.

The economics of laparoscopic colectomy

To date, all data suggest that laparoscopic colectomy takes significantly longer to perform than does open colectomy. The resultant increased operating room costs are likely responsible for the lack of significant savings in overall hospital charges to patients undergoing this procedure, as these patients may experience a shortened hospital stay. If operating room costs for laparoscopic colectomy can approximate those for open colectomy, there is likely to be a significant overall savings in health care cost.

Laparoscopic colon resection for malignant disease remains controversial. Experts have cautioned about the

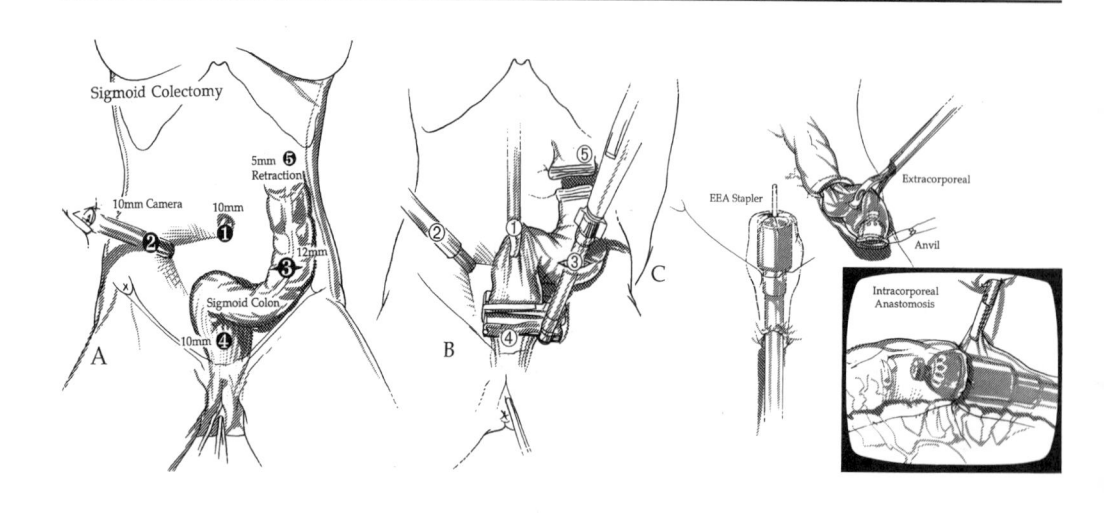

Fig. 3. Steps involved in sigmoid colectomy. (A) One suggested port placement. The port for the telescope and camera (no. 2) is placed in the right abdomen. Ports for the surgeon's left (no. 1) and right (no. 4) hands, as well as two ports for the assistant to retract and expose (nos. 3 and 5) are placed according to the segment of colon to be resected. (B) Site of port no. 3 used for placement of the roticulated TA-type stapler to perform distal bowel division in a case where low anterior resection is needed. (C) Anvil of the EEA-type circular stapler placed into the proximal end of the colon extracorporeally using the left lower quadrant incision. Shaft of the circular stapler advanced through the stapled end of the rectum in preparation for intracorporeal anastomosis (shown in insert).

Efficacy of right and segmental sigmoid resection for cancer

unbridled use of this procedure without appropriate evidence that surgical treatment of the tumor will not be compromised. Our own experience, as well as results reported by others,[5] suggests that the number of lymph nodes resected laparoscopically is similar to that traditionally removed with open celiotomy for certain segmental colectomies. Our experience has confirmed the efficacy of laparoscopic right and segmental sigmoid colon resection for cancer, as judged by histologic data and clear intraoperative visualization of the appropriate landmarks for boundaries of resection. Experience with resection of other segments of the colon has been more limited, and no preliminary impressions can be formulated. It should be emphasized that the optimal candidates for laparoscopic colon resections are those at high risk of the potential complications of a large open celiotomy incision, including patients with pulmonary insufficiency, obesity, or other medical problems that may increase perioperative morbidity, and who are counseled appropriately preoperatively.

Summary

Still experimental

Laparoscopic colon resection, despite encouraging preliminary results, should be evaluated further and performed only in situations where the experience will contribute objective data to the literature or to a registry where large numbers will have greater significance (such as the registry currently set up by the Society of Colon and Rectal Surgery). Further immediate evaluation of the safety and efficacy of the technique is indicated, especially as it relates to transverse colon resection, left hemicolectomy, abdominoperineal resection, and total colectomy. Further information is required regarding the steepness and extent of the learning curve for performing the procedure, and long-term follow-up is needed for patients undergoing laparoscopic colectomy for the management of carcinoma. Finally, laparoscopic colon resection should be attempted only by surgeons skilled in advanced laparoscopic surgical techniques, including mastery of the basics of two-handed dissection, laparoscopic exposure and retraction of viscera, and intracorporeal suturing and knot-tying.

LAPAROSCOPIC APPENDECTOMY

Laparoscopic appendectomy was first described by Semm in the early 1980s.[6] Initial acceptance was limited due to a low prevalence of laparoscopic skills among general surgeons who managed appendicitis. Until recently, the role of laparoscopy as reported in the literature was confined to diagnostic confirmation in cases of suspected acute appendicitis.[7,8] The emergence of laparoscopic cholecystectomy in the past 2 to 3 years has created an interest among general surgeons in performing appendectomy via a laparoscopic approach.

Indications

A most accurate diagnostic procedure

Laparoscopy offers the most accurate means of diagnosing acute appendicitis. Traditionally, the diagnosis of this condition has been a clinical one, based on a patient's history, physical findings, and laboratory findings. A misdiagnosis rate of 10% to 20% had been well accepted because the morbidity associated with an appendectomy in a normal patient was felt to be relatively low whereas the morbidity resulting from a missed case of acute appendicitis, with its progression to perforation and peritonitis, was considered substantial; for patients in some age groups it could even lead to death.[9]

The accuracy of diagnosing acute appendicitis based on the aforementioned criteria is often even lower, especially in the elderly and the very young. Some published reports have shown the incidence of misdiagnosis of acute appendicitis to approach 40% in women of menstruating age.[10] On the other hand, published data have reported the accuracy of diagnosing acute appendicitis by laparoscopy to be 95% or better in experienced hands.[7,8] This makes laparoscopy the procedure of choice for many patients suspected of having acute appendicitis. Laparoscopy allows the negative appendectomy rate to be lowered to 1%, while simultaneously allowing early and rapid diagnosis and treatment of acute appendicitis. Equally important is the fact that in the absence of acute appendicitis laparoscopy increases the incidence of correctly diagnosing right lower quadrant pain.

More appropriate for adolescents and adults

It has been argued that in patients less than 8 to 10 years of age the size of the incision required for appendectomy is similar to that required for laparoscopy. This, combined with the limitations of performing laparoscopy in the very small patient, may limit the application of laparoscopic appendectomy in children. However, laparoscopic appendectomy would seem to provide significantly better diagnostic accuracy in adolescents and adults.

Data regarding the therapeutic efficacy of laparoscopic appendectomy compared with traditional open appendectomy are still being gathered in meaningful form through prospective randomized trials. However, results of experiences to date suggest that the procedure can be performed safely and with good results in experienced hands.

Indications for conversion to open surgery

Although laparoscopy is frequently used to facilitate the diagnosis of appendicitis in adolescents and adults, there are certain patients in whom conversion from laparoscopy to open celiotomy is indicated, because of a severe inflammatory process, tissue quality, exposure, or other factors. As with laparoscopic cholecystectomy, the surgeon should not view this as a complication, but rather as good judgment in order to maximize patient safety and optimize the overall treatment results. The average conversion rate for appendectomy has not been determined, but will almost certainly decrease as surgical experience develops.

Patients with appendiceal abscess, in whom a mass is present but no signs of generalized peritonitis exist, may be managed initially with intravenous antibiotics alone. This situation suggests a contained perforation and localized abscess. Operative or percutaneous drainage followed by interval appendectomy after 2 to 3 months is associated with less morbidity than is initial operative appendectomy with disruption and drainage of the abscess.[11] We have successfully used two laparoscopic procedures for managing this condition: the first to confirm the diagnosis and guide drain placement, and the second to perform interval appendectomy.

Method of Laparoscopic Appendectomy

Operative principles for the management of uncomplicated appendicitis include proper preoperative preparation, administration of parenteral broad-spectrum antibiotics for enteric flora, good exposure and visualization of the appen-

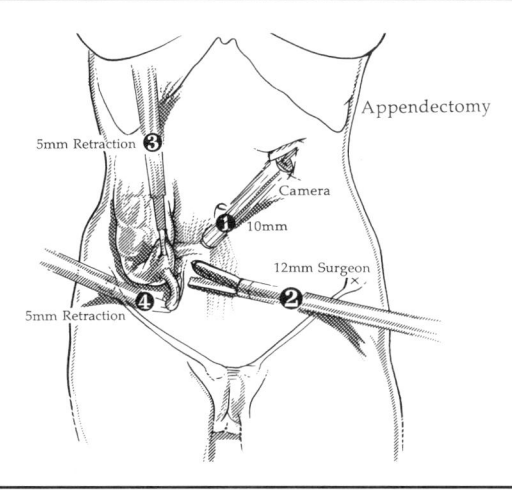

Fig. 4. Recommended port placement for laparoscopic appendectomy. The 10-mm umbilical port (no. 1) is used for the camera. A 12-mm port (no. 2) is placed in the left lower quadrant, allowing use of the endoscopic stapler. Two 5-mm ports (nos. 3 and 4) are used for appendiceal retraction and exposure.

dix, and secure ligation of the appendiceal mesentery and stump. Laparoscopic appendectomy allows all of these principles to be satisfied and also permits excellent inspection of the abdominal viscera for other potential problems should appendicitis not be found.

Laparoscopic appendectomy begins with the safe establishment of a pneumoperitoneum. Use of a Hasson trocar and open laparoscopy are indicated if the patient has undergone abdominal surgery previously or significant peritonitis and the potential for adhesions is present. Four ports are usually employed for laparoscopic appendectomy (Fig. 4), but three may be used. The umbilical port is for the telescope, and the right upper quadrant port is for retraction of the cecum or appendix. The suprapubic or left lower quadrant port is for dissection and ligation of the appendix and its mesentery. This can be a 10- or 12-mm port, depending on whether the endoscopic stapler, which requires a 12-mm trocar, is used. The optional but helpful fourth port is placed below the appendix, just above the inguinal ligament.

Semm[12] described the technique of laparoscopic appendectomy using Roeder loops to ligate the appendix (Fig. 5). Two loops are placed on the proximal stump of the appendix, with a single distal loop used to secure the divided stump. Sharp division of the appendix is recommended, as division by electrocautery could compromise the security of the proximal ties.

The mesentery to the appendix, including the appendiceal artery, must be secured to ensure good hemostasis. This may

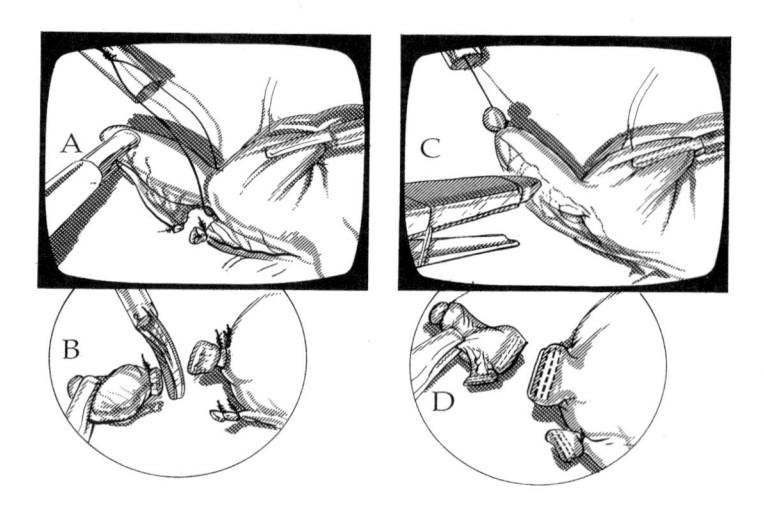

Fig. 5. Steps in laparoscopic appendectomy. (A) Division of the mesoappendix using Roeder loops or suture ligatures, followed by placement of two proximal and one distal Roeder loops on the appendix itself. (B) Sharp division of the appendix between ligatures. (C) Use of the vascular stapler to divide the mesoappendix. (D) Appendectomy completed after use of both vascular and intestinal staple loads of the endoscopic stapler.

be accomplished with suture ligatures, placed and tied intracorporeally, as advocated by Semm. Alternatively, vascular clips may be used. The vascular endoscopic stapler is another alternative, which we favor because of the security of its vascular ligation and the facility of its use. Inspection of the staple line is always necessary. If hemostasis is not complete, additional suture ligatures are placed and tied intracorporeally to secure any bleeding points. Although it is more expensive, the endoscopic stapler actually may be cost-effective when one considers the savings in operative time from using it to divide both the appendix (cartridge with 3.5-mm staples) and mesentery (cartridge with 2.5-mm staples).

Results of Laparoscopic Appendectomy

The largest series of laparoscopic appendectomies reported in the literature is by Gotz et al[13] from Germany. In 388 cases of appendicitis managed largely by laparoscopy, the complication rate was <1% and the rate of conversion to open celiotomy for completion of the operation was only 3%. An additional 7% of patients in this series had traditional celiotomy performed initially due to suspected perforation. That clinic has reported continued similarly impressive results with a series of 625 cases,[14] and other authors have reported success with laparoscopic appendectomy in a large series of children.[15]

Author's experience with laparoscopic appendectomy

Experience with laparoscopic appendectomy has been more limited in the United States than in Europe, where the procedure is established. Molnar et al[16] reported no significant decrease in the length of hospitalization for patients undergoing laparoscopic versus open appendectomy. Although no controlled randomized prospective trials have yet been published to address this issue, one is currently in progress in the United States. Hopefully, meaningful data will be available soon. The European experience suggests that laparoscopic appendectomy reduces in-hospital recovery time and time to return to normal activity.

We have found that laparoscopic appendectomy is associated with a significantly decreased incidence of wound infection.[17] This is important, as the average wound infection rate is 4% following negative appendectomies, 6% to 7% for nonperforated appendicitis, and 17.5% for perforated appendicitis.

Another advantage of laparoscopic appendectomy is the ability to correctly diagnose the source of abdominal inflammation at the time of surgery when acute appendicitis is not present.

Incidental Appendectomy

Incidental appendectomy is indicated for young patients still at significant risk of developing appendicitis. Complications of the procedure and operative costs outweigh the risks of potential appendicitis in patients over the age of 50 years.[18] It is unlikely that laparoscopic incidental appendectomy will be used extensively until it can be performed rapidly and safely enough to make it cost-effective for younger patients, as incidental appendectomy is currently performed during celiotomy at present. No data exist regarding the efficacy of incidental appendectomy during laparoscopy.

Summary

Laparoscopy appears to be of clear benefit in correctly diagnosing acute appendicitis. Laparoscopic appendectomy may hold certain advantages over traditional appendectomy for managing acute appendicitis, including lowering the incidence of wound infection. Whether laparoscopic appendectomy should become the treatment of choice for patients with suspected acute appendicitis awaits data from further studies.

OTHER INTESTINAL SURGERY

Table 3

Table 3 lists other intestinal procedures that can be and have been performed using laparoscopic techniques. Laparoscopic colostomy or ileostomy can be performed easily. The segment of bowel to be used for the stoma is mobilized suf-

Table 3. Other Laparoscopic Colon Procedures and Their Indications

Procedure	Indication
Diverting colostomy	Fecal incontinence Perineal wound Obstructing carcinoma Obstructing diverticulitis Trauma
Diverting ileostomy	Colonic anastomosis/leak Colonic inertia Obstructing Crohn's disease Obstructing carcinoma
Ripstein procedure	Rectal prolapse
Colostomy takedown	Presence of colostomy no longer indicated
Ileostomy takedown	Presence of ileostomy no longer indicated

ficiently by laparoscopy. A vessel loop is then passed around the bowel as would be done in the step to suspend the colon for segmental resection. However, the vessel loop is used as a guide to help pull the bowel gently through an appropriately large defect made in the abdomen directly above the mobilized bowel, allowing creation of the colostomy or ileostomy. Use of a TA-type stapler across the distal limb of the bowel results in a totally diverting stoma. We have used this procedure six times with good results at our institution.

Ileostomy or colostomy takedown does not require laparoscopic techniques where a loop stoma or the above stapled loop technique is used. However, in cases where a colostomy or ileostomy and Hartmann's procedure have been performed, laparoscopic dissection of the rectal or rectosigmoid stump can be instituted. Assistance from intraoperative proctoscopy or sigmoidoscopy can help define this segment of bowel. The stoma is taken down and the mobilized end of the proximal bowel is used for insertion of the anvil end of a circular stapling device secured with a purse-string suture. Transanal circular stapling of the bowel is then performed under laparoscopic guidance, as for low anterior resection.

Laparoscopy has been used to perform a Ripstein procedure for rectal prolapse.[19] The sling of prosthetic material is stapled or sutured to the presacral fascia for fixation.

Laparoscopic techniques used to perform small bowel resection are similar to those used for segmental colon resection. Intraoperative endoscopic localization of a mucosal intraluminal lesion is more limited in this setting, but many indications for small bowel resection involve pathology that is obvious to external examination of the intestine. The technique has been shown to be successful in the laboratory,[5] but reports of successful small bowel resection using laparoscopic techniques in patients are limited.

Successful laparoscopic-assisted resection of Meckel's diverticulum has been reported.[20] Laparoscopy was used to mobilize the diverticulum externally, with an external stapled resection being performed. This technique can now be performed intracorporeally, using the endoscopic stapler.

In all of these additional procedures, initial clinical observations have suggested that laparoscopy affords the benefits of limiting incision size, lessening postoperative pain, and minimizing wound complications, as is true for laparoscopic cholecystectomy. However, data to support this contention are limited.

References
1. Jacobs M, et al. *Surg Laparosc Endosc* 1991;1:144-150.
2. Cooperman AM, et al. *J Laparoendosc Surg* 1991;1:221-224.
3. Redwine DB, Sharpe DR. *J Laparoendosc Surg* 1991;1:217-220.
4. Wexner SD, et al. *Dis Colon Rectum* 1992;35:651-665.
5. *Advanced Laparoscopic Bowel/Colon & Rectal Seminar* (syllabus). Ethicon Corporation, Endo-Surgery Institute, Cincinnati, Ohio, 1992.
6. Semm K. *Endoscopy* 1983;15:59-64.
7. Leape LL, Ramenofsky ML. *Ann Surg* 1980;191:410-413.
8. Whitworth CM, et al. *Surg Gynecol Obstet* 1988;167:187-190.
9. Lewis FR, et al. *Arch Surg* 1975;110:677-684.
10. Chang FC, et al. *Am J Surg* 1973;126:752-754.
11. Skoubo-Kristensen E, Hvid I. *Ann Surg* 1982;196:584-587.
12. Semm K. *Pelviscopy–Operative Guideline*. New York, NY, Year Book Medical Publishers, 1987.
13. Gotz F, et al. *Surg Endosc* 1990;4:6.
14. Pier A, et al. *Surg Laparosc Endosc* 1991;1:8.
15. Valla JS, et al. *Surg Laparosc Endosc* 1991;1:166-172.
16. Molnar RG, Apelgren KN. *Is Laparoscopic Better Than Open Appendectomy?* Presented at the Society of Gastrointestinal Endoscopic Surgeons Scientific Session, Washington, DC, April 1992.
17. Schirmer BD, et al. *Laparoscopic Versus Traditional Appendectomy for Suspected Appendicitis*. Presented at the 33rd Annual Meeting of the Society for Surgery of the Alimentary Tract. San Francisco, Calif, May 1992.
18. Nockerts SR, et al. *Surgery* 1980;88:301-306.
19. Kuminsky RE, et al. *Surg Laparosc Endosc* 1992;2:346-347.
20. Attwood SEA, et al. *Br J Surg* 1992;79:211.

III Laparoscopic Treatment of Gallstones

Nathaniel J. Soper, MD

BRIEF CONTENTS	Introduction	38
	Preoperative Considerations	40
	Indications	40
	Contraindications	41
	Equipment	41
	Preoperative Care and Anesthesia	44
	Creation of a Pneumoperitoneum and Trocar Insertion	45
	The Closed Technique	46
	The Open Technique	48
	Technique of Laparoscopic Cholecystectomy	49
	Special Considerations in the Performance of Laparoscopic Cholecystectomy	58
	Anatomic Hazards	58
	Conversion to Open Operation	59
	Acute Cholecystitis	60
	Intraoperative Gallbladder Perforation	61

BRIEF CONTENTS (continued)

Cholangiography	61
Complications of Laparoscopic Cholecystectomy	62
Postoperative Care	65
Results of Laparoscopic Cholecystectomy	65
Author's Personal Series	65
Other Reported Series	66
Results of the National Institutes of Health Consensus Development Conference	67
Management of Common Bile Duct Stones	68
Conclusion	71

INTRODUCTION

The first laparoscopic cholecystectomy was performed in 1985 by Mühe[1] of Böblingen, Germany; however, many authors have assigned this credit to Mouret[2] of Lyon, France, who performed a similar procedure in 1987. The procedure was facilitated by rotating the entire right lobe of the liver cephalad and by applying traction to the gallbladder itself. This allowed the gallbladder and porta hepatis to be viewed from a telescope placed at the umbilicus and directed cranially toward the undersurface of the liver. Surgeons in Paris and Bordeaux, France subsequently learned the procedure, and thus began the early clinical series of laparoscopic cholecystectomies.[2,3] In mid-1988 this procedure was first performed in the United States and has since been reported by Reddick and Olsen[4,5] and many others.[6-13] Because of the competitive free-market medical system that prevails in the United States, the preference by patients for less invasive procedures, and the marketing efforts of individuals and hospitals, laparoscopic cholecystectomy has been adopted at a rate unprecedented in American surgery.

The explosion of interest in this operation is reflected by events at the last few meetings of the American College of Surgeons. At the trade exhibits in Atlanta in 1989 there were two videotapes of laparoscopic cholecystectomy available for

Rapid adoption of laparoscopic cholecystectomy by American surgeons and public

Table 1. Comparison of Laparoscopic Cholecystectomy With Other Therapies for Cholelithiasis

Comparative Procedure	Laparoscopic Cholecystectomy	
	Advantages	Disadvantages
Nonresective Therapies	Removal of diseased gallbladder Minimal chance of gallstone recurrence Few exclusion criteria	Patients must be candidates for general anesthesia Higher morbidity and mortality
Open Cholecystectomy	Smaller incisions Less pain Shorter hospitalization More rapid return to full activity Decreased total cost	Technical limitations: More difficult to control hemorrhage and explore common bile duct; monocular vision controlled by assistant; expensive, technologically advanced instruments required Anatomical limitations: Inflammation/adhesions restrict application; difficult antegrade removal of gallbladder; possibly increased incidence of bile duct injury

Advantages

Table 1

viewing but no mention of the procedure in the scientific program. At the trade exhibits in San Francisco in 1990 laparoscopic surgery was presented in at least 50 of the trade booths, 15 of the scientific exhibits, two full afternoons of audiovisual cine-clinics, a paper on the plenary session, and a postgraduate course. It has been reported that more than 25,000 general surgeons have been trained in laparoscopic cholecystectomy since 1989.[14]

There are many potential advantages of laparoscopic cholecystectomy over other therapies for cholelithiasis (Table 1)[15]: (1) The diseased gallbladder is removed along with its stones, in contrast to the nonresective techniques for gallstone ablation; (2) postoperative pain and intestinal ileus are diminished in comparison with traditional open cholecystectomy; (3) the small size of the fascial incisions allows a rapid return to heavy physical activities; (4) the multiple small incisions are cosmetically more appealing than is the large incision made during traditional cholecystectomy; and (5) patients usually can be discharged from the hospital on the day of surgery or the day following, and can return to full activity within a few days.[16] These factors have led to a reduced overall cost of the procedure.[17,18] However, there are

Table 2. Contraindications to Laparoscopic Cholecystectomy

Absolute	Relative
Inability to tolerate general anesthesia	Acute cholecystitis with suspected empyema
Uncorrected coagulopathy	Morbid obesity
Peritonitis/cholangitis	Previous upper abdominal surgery
Biliary fistula	Cirrhosis/portal hypertension
Suspected carcinoma	Severe obstructive lung disease
	Pregnancy

Disadvantages

several disadvantages of laparoscopic cholecystectomy, as well: (1) Patients must be acceptable candidates for general anesthesia; (2) three-dimensional depth perception is limited by the monocular image of the video telescope, and the operative field being viewed is determined by an individual other than the surgeon; (3) some patients may be excluded from undergoing this therapy because of their anatomy or intra-abdominal adhesions; (4) the common bile duct is more difficult to visualize and to instrument with laparoscopic techniques than during traditional open surgery; and (5) it is technically difficult to remove the gallbladder from the fundus to the infundibulum and more difficult to control brisk hemorrhage using laparoscopic techniques than in an open surgical field. In the ensuing discussion, the current status of the laparoscopic management of gallstones will be reviewed, focusing on preoperative, intraoperative, and postoperative considerations.

PREOPERATIVE CONSIDERATIONS
Indications

The ability to perform laparoscopic cholecystectomy should not expand the indications for removing the gallbladder. In general, patients should have documented cholelithiasis and symptoms of gallbladder disease. Occasionally, individuals with gallstones and no symptoms (eg, patients with a porcelain gallbladder, immunosuppressed patients, patients whose life-styles remove them from access to medical care) or those with no gallstones but typical biliary symptoms (eg, documented biliary dyskinesia) may be considered for this therapy. Recent studies suggest that less than 20% of individuals with asymptomatic gallstones develop symptoms over a prolonged period, and that the risk of prophylactic surgery outweighs its potential benefit.[19,20]

In an individual with typical biliary colic, the only diagnostic test necessary is high-quality ultrasound. This study demonstrates the size and number of the stones, the thickness of the gallbladder wall, and the diameter of the common bile duct. It also may suggest nonbiliary disorders such as hepatic lesions or fatty infiltration, masses in the pancreas, and renal tumors. If atypical symptoms are present, a more extensive work-up may be appropriate. This includes upper gastrointestinal contrast radiography or endoscopy, computerized tomography, and cardiac evaluation.

Contraindications

Table 2

The contraindications to laparoscopic cholecystectomy have changed tremendously as experience has grown with this technique. Absolute contraindications and numerous relative contraindications dictated primarily by the surgeon's philosophy and experience are listed in Table 2. Many of these relative contraindications were once considered absolute contraindications. Certainly, it would be wise for the novice laparoscopic surgeon to avoid patients with such contraindications for his or her first few procedures. Despite scattered reports of laparoscopic cholecystectomies having been performed on pregnant women,[21] the effects of the prolonged carbon dioxide pneumoperitoneum on the fetus are unknown, and the position of the gravid uterus itself may present a problem.

Equipment

Required equipment for basic laparoscopy

The equipment necessary for basic laparoscopy includes a machine to insufflate the abdomen with gas, a fiber-optic light source to transmit light to the interior of the abdomen, a telescope to transmit an image to the external surface, and a gasketed laparoscopic sheath to maintain access to the abdominal cavity without allowing excessive gas to escape. For therapeutic laparoscopy, the insufflator should be capable of delivering at least 6 L/min of the appropriate gas (usually carbon dioxide), maintain the pressure at a preset level, and terminate insufflation when the desired pressure limit has been reached. Adequate light for therapeutic procedures is afforded by a xenon light source.

The laparoscope

Laparoscopes come in various sizes, but usually are 5 or 10 mm in diameter and can be end-viewing (0°) or have an angled lens on the tip (30° or 45° forward-oblique). The end-viewing telescope transmits more light and is easier to use; the view is less distorted and the radial orientation of the scope itself does not influence the image. The oblique-viewing telescope is valuable for looking around corners, which can help assess the anterior abdominal wall, the dome of the liver, and the extremities of the abdominal cavity. A number of companies are developing three-dimensional laparoscopic systems as well as flexible laparoscopes, which may play a significant role in the future.

Therapeutic laparoscopy is almost always performed with a video camera harnessed to the eyepiece of the laparoscope, which transmits the image to a video screen. It is useful to have video monitors on each side of the operating table so that the surgeon and assistant may stand on opposite sides of the table while viewing the same image comfortably. Documentation of the procedure is facilitated by a video recorder.

Trocars and sheaths

Various laparoscopic trocars and sheaths are available. They range from 3 to 15 mm in diameter and must be 0.5 mm larger than the instruments that will be placed through them. The sheaths may be reusable or disposable, radiolucent or radiopaque. The reusable sheaths are equipped with rotational valves or trumpet valves, and conical or pyramidal trocars for puncturing the abdominal wall, and contain gaskets to prevent gas leak. Disposable surgical trocar/sheath assemblies have been designed by a number of manufacturers. These instruments are always sharp, have more dependable gaskets to prevent gas leak, and often are radiolucent. The disposable ports incorporate a retractable safety shield that covers the trocar point following entry into the abdomen. This helps prevent trauma to the internal viscera but does not guarantee protection of the underlying viscera because of sheath drag through the abdominal wall, whereby there is a finite period during which the trocar blade is exposed upon entry through the peritoneum. Of note, these disposable instruments are relatively expensive.

Laparoscopic cholecystectomy sets

For laparoscopic cholecystectomy, most American surgeons use two large (10- or 11-mm) and two small (5-mm) trocar/sheath assemblies. Various instruments can then be used to perform the actual operation, and most manufacturers now sell laparoscopic cholecystectomy instrument sets. These sets include forceps designed to grasp the gallbladder without puncturing it and extract the gallbladder through the incision at the end of the operation. A number of dissecting instruments are available with jaw designs whose surface contours and angulations vary markedly depending on the intended use. Laparoscopic scissors come in different sizes and tip designs, also depending on the intended use. For laparoscopic suturing, there are numerous 3- and 5-mm needle holders with differing jaw designs and handle configurations, from handles oriented at right angles to the shaft to coaxial handles. Most contain ratcheted locking jaws.

Most surgeons use cautery rather than lasers to transmit thermal energy to the interior of the abdomen for hemostasis. Monopolar or bipolar cautery can be applied with various spatula- and hook-tipped probes. Many of these probes are hollow to allow for the irrigation and aspiration of small volumes of fluid. For more active peritoneal lavage, a number

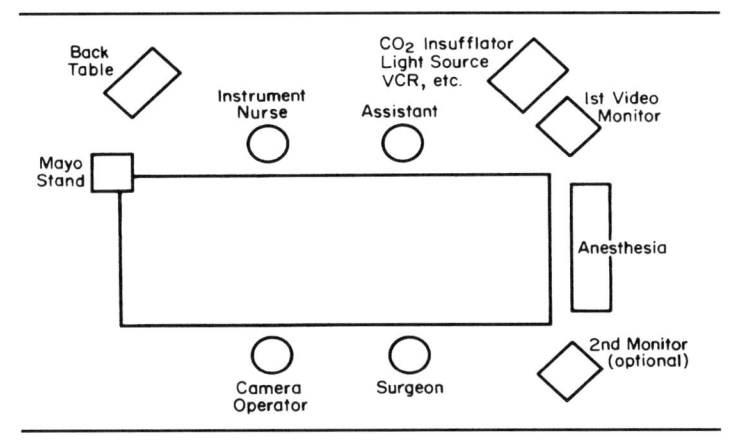

Fig. 1. Organization of the operating room for laparoscopic biliary surgery. The patient's head is to the right, the surgeon stands at the patient's left, and the first assistant stands to the patient's right. The electronic laparoscopic equipment is placed on protective carts, and the monitors are positioned to allow clear visualization by the entire surgical team. (From Soper NJ.[15] Reproduced with permission.)

of suction-irrigation probes are available that may infuse irrigant at a rate of up to 10 L/min. For occluding the cystic duct and artery most surgeons use a laparoscopic clip applier. Clip appliers may be reusable and manually loaded or disposable, automated, and preloaded with a number of clips of varying lengths. Advantages of the disposable clip appliers include rapidity of use and avoidance of multiple entries through the laparoscopic sheaths.

For manipulation of common bile duct stones various instruments may be desirable. These include guide wires, balloon dilators, multiwired expandable baskets for stone extraction, and small flexible choledochoscopes (usually a modification of the 8- to 10-F ureteroscope).

Finally, any surgeon performing laparoscopic cholecystectomy should have a standard cholecystectomy set available. The surgeon should be able to expose the gallbladder bed within seconds should the need arise. We routinely keep a scalpel, four Kelly clamps, two Army/Navy retractors, Kocher clamps, a curved Mayo scissors, and 1-0 and 4-0 gauge sutures sterile on the back table.

Operating room setup

The equipment necessary to perform laparoscopic cholecystectomy is bulky, expensive, and technologically advanced. The video monitor need go blank only once to remind the operator how dependent he or she is on the equipment. The electronic equipment should be placed on carts to protect and organize it into a unit. We set up our operating room for laparoscopic biliary surgery as shown in Fig. 1. The equipment must be handled carefully, and skilled personnel are necessary for maintenance. The forceps and other laparoscopic instruments are delicate and break easily.

Figure 1

Positioning of personnel

A biomedical engineer or a trained technician must be available to correct any electronic problems that arise. Finally, appropriate safeguards must be put in place to protect the patient during the laparoscopic cholecystectomy. Due to the frequent repositioning of the table, the patient must be strapped in place and a foot board used. If a laser is employed, the eyes of the patient and operating room personnel should be covered with appropriate eyewear. The electrocautery unit must be grounded following standard protocol and calibrated at intervals suggested by the manufacturer. Finally, as the light source may become hot, the scope end of the light cable must be covered to protect the patient and staff from burns.

Laparoscopic biliary surgery requires more personnel than do open operations. The surgeon stands to the left of the patient for cross-table access to the right upper quadrant (Fig. 1). The first assistant stands to the patient's right to manipulate the gallbladder and provide exposure. A trained laparoscopic video camera operator stands below the surgeon and assumes the important responsibility of being the surgeon's eyes. The camera operator must maintain the proper orientation of the camera, keep the surgeon's instruments in the center of the video monitor, follow or guide all of the instruments as they enter or exit the operative field, and assist with the grasping forceps or trumpet valves as needed. No sharp instruments should be moved unless they can be visualized directly. Likewise, the camera operator must remove any visual obstruction (eg, wipe condensation or blood from the lens). Condensation on the lens itself can be minimized by heating the laparoscope prior to its insertion into the warm, moist abdominal cavity.

PREOPERATIVE CARE AND ANESTHESIA

As for any abdominal operation, patients are fasted from midnight prior to the day of surgery. Patients without other major medical problems are admitted to the hospital on the morning of surgery and receive preoperative sedatives. All patients are administered intravenous broad-spectrum antibiotics prophylactically. When the patient arrives in the operating room, sequential compression stockings are placed on both legs to avoid pooling of blood in the lower extremities caused by the reverse Trendelenburg position. We have not routinely used mini-dose heparin, but this can be administered safely to patients at risk of venous thromboembolism. After the induction of anesthesia, a bladder catheter and orogastric tube are placed to decompress the hollow organs. The abdomen is prepared in standard fashion, but particular care is taken to clean the umbilicus of all detritus.

Inhalation anesthesia

Although diagnostic laparoscopy can be performed using local or regional anesthesia, laparoscopic cholecystectomy is generally performed using inhalation anesthesia and controlled ventilation. Important considerations for optimal anesthetic management include (1) adequate depth of anesthesia; (2) complete muscle relaxation; (3) the administration of amnesics; and (4) the administration of an antiemetic prior to the conclusion of surgery. Appropriate patient monitoring during therapeutic laparoscopy using general anesthesia includes electrocardiography, blood pressure measurement, precordial stethoscopy, airway pressure measurement, and capnography (specifically to assess end-tidal carbon dioxide). Invasive monitoring by means of an arterial line and Swan-Ganz catheter may be indicated in selected high-risk individuals.[22,23]

There have been scattered reports of laparoscopic cholecystectomy performed using thoracic epidural (bupivacaine) anesthesia supplemented with intravenous sedation and local anesthesia. Referred shoulder pain may be troublesome when this technique is used, but the pain may be diminished by insufflating the peritoneal cavity slowly and by maintaining a lower abdominal pressure (<10 mm Hg). Regional anesthesia may be appropriate for high-risk patients or those who are highly motivated to avoid a general anesthetic. However, the potential need for rapid conversion to an open laparotomy has led us to use general anesthesia in all cases.

CREATION OF A PNEUMOPERITONEUM AND TROCAR INSERTION

Elevation of the abdomen for visualization

The establishment of a pneumoperitoneum by the instillation of gas permits visualization of the abdominal cavity. Devices that elevate the abdominal wall by external retraction have been described recently,[24] and ultimately may replace peritoneal insufflation for abdominal wall lift during laparoscopy. For diagnostic laparoscopy carbon dioxide and nitrous oxide are applicable. Although it is nonflammable, nitrous oxide supports combustion and, therefore, is not usually used for creating the pneumoperitoneum for laparoscopic cholecystectomy. Carbon dioxide has the advantage of being noncombustible and rapidly absorbable from the peritoneal cavity; most carbon dioxide disappears within 4 hours of the conclusion of surgery. It is absorbed readily into the blood stream and may lead to hypercarbia in patients with chronic obstructive pulmonary disease. Because the gas is converted to carbonic acid on the moist peritoneal surface it may cause mild discomfort postoperatively. Absorption of carbon dioxide from the blood is rapid; the body can safely absorb carbon dioxide when infused into a systemic vein at a rate of <1 L/min.[25]

The pneumoperitoneum can be established by a closed or

an open technique. With the closed technique carbon dioxide is insufflated into the peritoneal cavity through a needle after which the initial laparoscopic trocar and sheath are placed blindly into the abdominal cavity. With the open technique a small incision is made and a laparoscopic sheath without the sharp trocar is inserted under direct vision into the peritoneal cavity. Only after ensuring safe peritoneal entry is the pneumoperitoneum established. There are advantages and disadvantages to both techniques, and surgeons performing laparoscopy should be familiar with both and use them on a selective basis.

The Closed Technique
Carbon dioxide is insufflated through a Veress needle or one of its disposable counterparts. Prior to insertion, the pneumoperitoneum needle should be checked to ensure that the spring-loaded stylet is functioning properly and that the lumen is patent to the injection of water. The patient is then placed in a 10° to 15° Trendelenburg position, and an examination is performed, with the patient under anesthesia, to assess the site of the aortic bifurcation. In the nonoperated abdomen the Veress needle and initial trocar are inserted into the infraumbilical skin fold. A small vertical or circumumbilical incision is made into the subcutaneous tissue. The surgeon stands to the left of the patient and grasps the lower abdomen with his or her left hand, elevating and stabilizing the abdominal wall. The Veress needle is then inserted at a right angle to the abdominal wall, usually 45° off the vertical axis toward the pelvis. The surgeon will hear one or two clicks of the obturator as the needle passes into the peritoneal cavity. Various tests to assure the safety of the needle insertion are then performed. A syringe containing normal saline solution, 5 mL, is attached to the Luer lock connector to aspirate and demonstrate the absence of blood, urine, or stool. If the aspiration is negative, it is repeated after the injection of a few milliliters of saline. If blood-stained fluid or frank blood is recovered the needle should be removed and its position changed. If no fluid is aspirated an assessment is made of the ease with which the saline flows by gravity into the relatively negative pressure of the peritoneal cavity. This is done by instilling a few drops of saline into the hub of the needle or removing the barrel of the syringe. Manually elevating the lower abdominal wall will decrease intra-abdominal pressure and enhance free flow; the fluid will flow much more slowly if the needle is in the preperitoneal space.

An alternative site for initial puncture may be required in patients who have undergone abdominal surgery previously. With an upper midline scar, the puncture should be made in the right or left lower quadrant two thirds of the distance

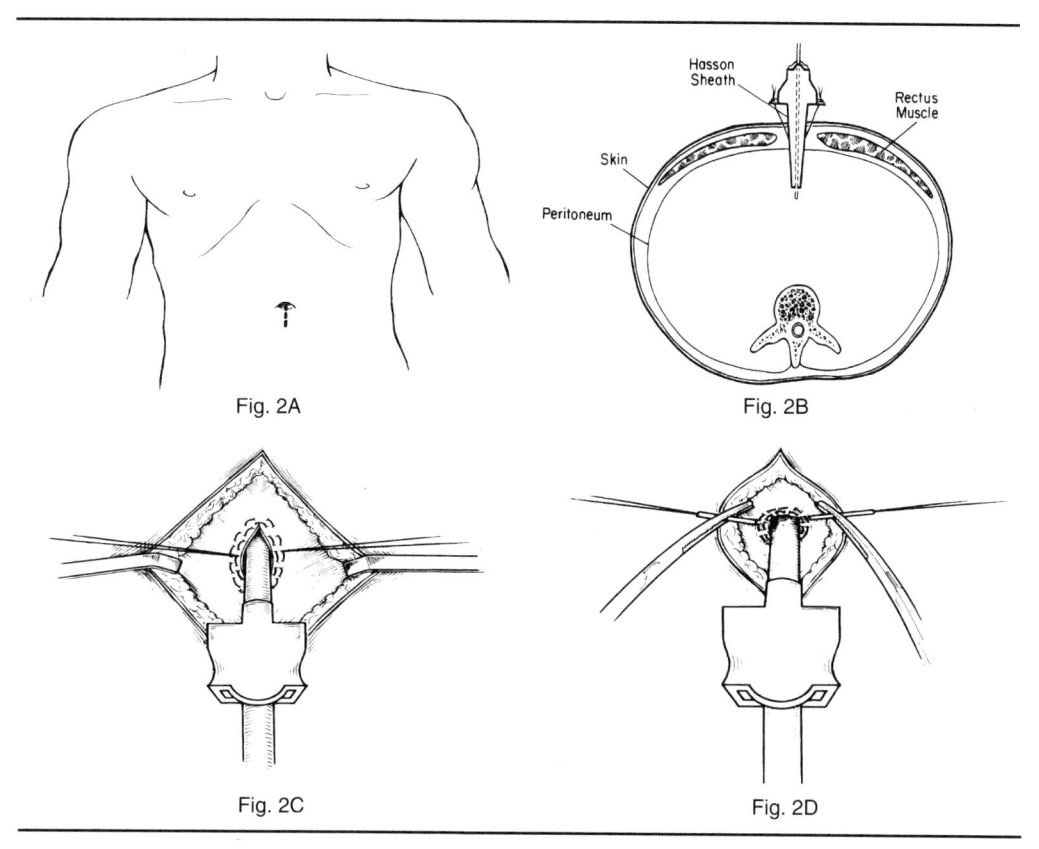

Fig. 2. Techniques for open insertion of the initial laparoscopic sheath. (A) Site of skin incision. (B) Placement of Hasson sheath through the abdominal wall and securement with sutures between the fascia and wings of the sheath. (C, D) Use of a standard laparoscopic sheath and two concentric purse-string sutures placed in the abdominal fascia as an alternative technique. (From Soper NJ.[15] Reproduced with permission.)

from the umbilicus to the iliac crest. A lower midline scar favors an initial puncture in the right or left upper abdomen at the lateral edge of the rectus muscle. If this approach is used, the position of the liver and spleen must be ascertained prior to needle insertion. The tubing from the insufflator is then connected to the Veress needle and carbon dioxide is insufflated at an initial rate of 1 L/min. The abdomen is percussed to confirm symmetric tympany associated with the intraperitoneal gas and then is inflated with the insufflator's upper pressure limit set at 15 mm Hg. This usually requires 3.5 to 6 L of carbon dioxide, depending on the size of the abdominal cavity and the weight of the abdominal wall. Patients who are obese or muscular tend to have heavier abdominal walls and higher abdominal pressures, and sometimes require an increased pressure limit to allow for an adequate pneumoperitoneum.

Monitoring for gas embolism

During the early phase of insufflation the patient must be monitored closely for signs of gas embolism (eg, hypotension, "millwheel" heart murmur), vagal reaction (eg, hypotension, bradycardia), ventricular arrhythmias, and hypercarbia with acidosis. Most of these complications require immediate treatment by allowing escape of the gas and gradually reestablishing the pneumoperitoneum after the patient's condition has stabilized. Gas embolism results in an "air-lock" right ventricular outflow obstruction. When this is suspected, the patient should be placed in the Trendelenburg position with the left side down and a central venous catheter inserted to aspirate the carbon dioxide. When the intra-abdominal pressure exceeds 20 mm Hg, central venous pressure and blood pressure fall in association with diminished cardiac output. Adequate muscle relaxation helps minimize the rise in intra-abdominal pressure. After the pneumoperitoneum has been established the Veress needle is removed.

The initial large (10- to 11-mm) trocar and sheath are placed in the infraumbilical incision created previously. They are inserted with a gentle drilling motion for controlled entry into the peritoneal cavity. The sheath is inserted at the same angle as the Veress needle while the lower abdominal wall is stabilized manually. With practice, it becomes apparent when the resistance of the fascia and peritoneum is overcome and the sheath enters the abdominal cavity. With a nondisposable trocar, the hissing noise of escaping carbon dioxide gas indicates that the trocar tip is positioned correctly in the pneumoperitoneal space. With a disposable sheath the safety shield can be heard springing into place over the trocar tip. The trocar is then removed and the telescope is inserted.

The Open Technique

Creation of the pneumoperitoneum by the open technique is similar to open diagnostic peritoneal lavage. A 1.5-cm vertical or horizontal skin incision is made in the infraumbilical skin fold (Fig. 2A). Subcutaneous tissue should be dissected deep to the skin of the umbilicus to reach the fascia quickly, even in obese patients, as this is the thinnest part of the abdominal wall. Kocher clamps are then applied to both sides of the midline of the linea alba, and a small vertical incision is made into the peritoneal cavity. A finger is placed into the wound to assure that the free peritoneal cavity has been entered and to sweep away any adhesions. If Hasson trocars are available, two heavy absorbable sutures are placed on both sides of the fascial incision and are tied to the wings of the olive-tipped trocar after its insertion into the peritoneal cavity under direct vision (Fig. 2B). Alternatively, standard laparoscopic sheaths can be used after placing two concentric purse-string stitches of heavy monofilament suture around the fascial

Figure 2A

Figure 2B

Figures 2C & 2D

incision (Figs. 2C,D). The laparoscopic sleeve without its sharp trocar is then inserted into the peritoneal cavity and the purse-string sutures are tightened down using a section of red rubber catheter similar to a vascular tourniquet. After removing the sheath, the outer purse-string suture is removed and the inner one is tied down. Open insertion of the initial port takes a few minutes longer than its closed counterpart. However, extraction of the gallbladder at the conclusion of the operation is easier. We perform open insertion of the sheath selectively: in patients with previous periumbilical incisions, patients in whom insertion of the Veress needle is not performed satisfactorily, and patients with large (>2.5 cm) gallstones or acute cholecystitis.

TECHNIQUE OF LAPAROSCOPIC CHOLECYSTECTOMY

A 10.5-mm laparoscope is inserted into the abdomen. The retroperitoneum immediately posterior to the umbilicus and the pelvis are viewed first to assure that there is no injury as a result of the insertion of the trocar or sheath. The pelvic viscera are examined for other pathologic abnormalities prior to evaluation of the upper abdomen. The anterior surfaces of the intestines, omentum, and stomach are examined for abnormalities. During this maneuver the patient is placed in a reverse Trendelenburg position of 30° to 40° as the table is rotated to the patient's left by 15° to 20°. This maneuver generally allows the colon and duodenum to fall away from the edge of the liver. The falciform ligament and both lobes of the liver are examined closely for abnormalities. The inferior margin of the liver is then visualized to determine the location of the gallbladder. Usually, the gallbladder can be seen protruding beyond the edge of the liver, but it may not be visible without careful elevation of the liver's right lobe.

Next, the two small accessory subcostal ports are placed under direct vision. The first trocar is placed in the anterior to middle axillary line between the 12th rib and the iliac crest. This sheath should be placed inferior (caudad) to the gallbladder fundus and liver edge. A second 5-mm port is then inserted under direct vision midway between the axillary sheath and the xiphoid process. Major abdominal wall blood vessels can be avoided during trocar insertion by a combination of transillumination and direct examination of the parietal peritoneum. Grasping forceps are then placed through these two sheaths and the gallbladder is secured. The assistant, standing on the right side of the table, manipulates the lateral grasping forceps used to elevate the liver edge to expose the fundus of the gallbladder. The surgeon, standing to the left of the patient, uses a dissecting forceps to raise a serosal fold of the most dependent portion of the fundus. The assistant's heavy grasping forceps are then

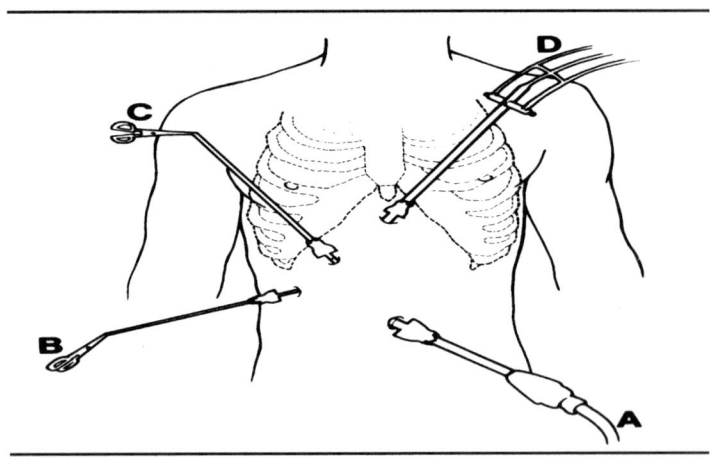

Fig. 3. Positions for insertion of the (A) initial and (B-D) accessory sheaths for biliary surgery. (From Soper NJ.[15] Reproduced with permission.)

locked onto this fold using a spring or ratchet device. With the axillary grasping forceps the fundus of the gallbladder is pushed laterally and cephalad, rolling the entire right lobe of the liver cranially. The successful performance of this maneuver is critical to expose the porta hepatis and gallbladder. The position of these trocars in patients with high- or low-lying livers is different than in the average patient. A fixed, cirrhotic liver or heavy, friable liver resulting from fatty infiltration will complicate this maneuver.

In patients with few gallbladder adhesions, pushing the fundus cephalad exposes the entire gallbladder, cystic duct, and porta hepatis. However, most patients have adhesions between the gallbladder and the omentum, hepatic flexure, and/or duodenum. Generally, these adhesions are avascular and may be lysed bluntly; this involves grasping them with a dissecting forceps at their site of attachment to the gallbladder wall and gently stripping them down toward the infundibulum. After the infundibulum is exposed, blunt grasping forceps are placed through the midclavicular trocar for traction on the neck of the gallbladder. The operative field is thereby established, and the final working port is then inserted.

The last 10- to 11-mm trocar is placed through a transverse incision in the midline of the epigastrium. Usually, this is placed 5 cm below the xiphoid process but the position depends on the location of the gallbladder as well as on the size of the medial segment of the left lobe of the liver. If the operator is uncertain about the appropriate position for this trocar, a Veress needle may be placed at the proposed site to ascertain whether its location and angle of insertion are optimal. Following this the trocar is inserted with a drilling

Figure 3

motion with its tip angled just to the right of the falciform ligament and aimed toward the gallbladder. An 11- to 5-mm laparoscopic reducer is then placed into the sheath, and a 5-mm dissecting forceps is inserted into the operative field.

The basic positions for placement of the various ports are shown in Fig. 3. The accessory sheaths should be separated as widely as possible so that the external portions of the instruments do not cross or interfere with each other. The orientation of the laparoscope is parallel to that of the cystic duct when the fundus is elevated; the instruments placed through the axillary and epigastric sheaths enter the abdomen at right angles to this plane. Finally, the midclavicular sheath is anterior to the gallbladder so that the instruments passing through it are perpendicular to the cystic duct. Thus, all of the accessory sheaths are placed at right angles to the axis of the cystic duct while the surgeon's vision is directed along its axis.

Having established the positions of all of the sheaths, the first assistant places the fundus and infundibulum of the gallbladder under tension away from the common bile duct in a superior and lateral direction. The surgeon then may use a one-handed dissection technique while working through the epigastric portal. The left hand is placed on the laparoscopic sheath to stabilize its position and regulate its gross movements. The right hand is placed on the dissecting instrument to control the fine motions of the tip of the instrument. However, many surgeons prefer using a two-handed technique, manipulating the infundibulum of the gallbladder with

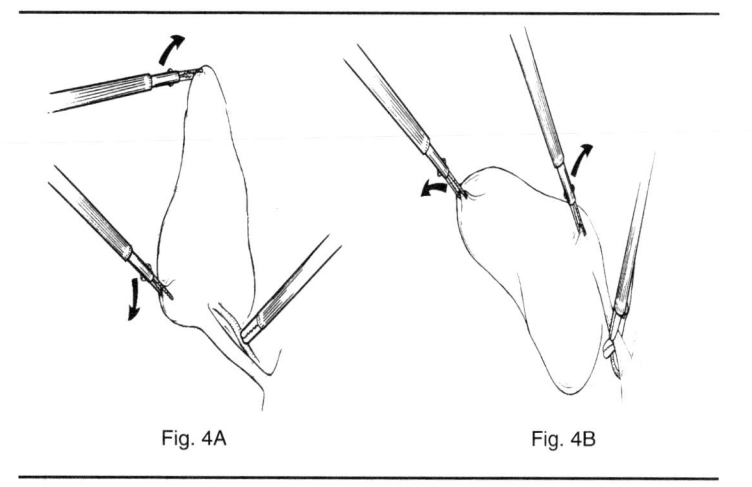

Fig. 4A   Fig. 4B

Fig. 4. (A) Calot's triangle, exposed by manipulation of the gallbladder with traction applied by the assistant's grasping forceps. The surgeon's curved instrument encirlces the cystic artery; the cystic duct is anterior. Arrows indicate vector of forceps movement. (B) The reverse (dorsal aspect) of Calot's triangle. Arrows indicate vector of forceps movement. (From Soper NJ.[15] Reproduced with permission.)

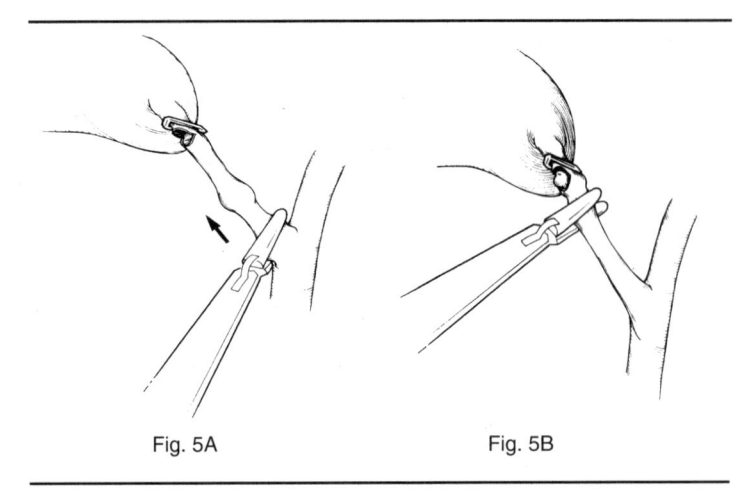

Fig. 5. (A) Gentle squeezing and (B) milking of the cystic duct toward the gallbladder to diagnose and remove cystic duct stones. (From Soper NJ, Dunnegan DL.[40] Reproduced with permission.)

Figure 4A

the left hand while performing dissection with instruments in the right hand. With the fundus and neck of the gallbladder under tension, a fine-tipped dissecting forceps is used to separate the overlying fibroareolar structures from the infundibulum of the gallbladder and Hartmann's pouch. This is done with a blunt stripping action, always starting on the gallbladder and pulling the tissue toward the porta hepatis. The dissection should begin on a known structure (eg, the gallbladder) rather than in an unknown area, to avoid damage to the bile duct or hepatic artery.

During this initial dissection around the neck of the gallbladder, the peritoneum is lysed with the blunt dissector. This technique is similar to that by which the peritoneum is incised and pushed bluntly with a Kittner dissector during traditional open cholecystectomy. With the laparoscopic dissection performed under two-dimensional optics, it is critical to clear and identify the structures contained within two triangles: Calot's triangle and the reverse side of Calot's triangle. Calot's triangle is the ventral aspect of the area bounded by the cystic duct, hepatic duct, and liver edge. The reverse side of Calot's triangle is the dorsal aspect of this space. Calot's triangle is placed on tension and exposed maximally by retracting the infundibulum of the gallbladder inferiorly and laterally while pushing the fundus superiorly and medially (Fig. 4A). A lymph node usually overlies the cystic artery; occasionally it is necessary to apply an electric current for a brief period to achieve hemostasis as the lymph node is swept away. The assistant then places the infundibulum of the gallbladder on stretch superiorly and medially

Figure 4B

while pushing the fundus superiorly and laterally, thereby exposing the reverse side of Calot's triangle, an area defined by the cystic duct, inferior lateral border of the gallbladder, and right lobe of the liver (Fig. 4B). Further blunt dissection is performed to identify precisely the junction between the infundibulum and the origin of the cystic duct. Identification of this junction is the critical maneuver in the operation; no structure should be sharply divided until the cystic duct is identified clearly. The strands of peritoneal, lymphatic, neural, and vascular tissue are stripped away from the cystic duct to gain as much length as possible. A curved dissecting forceps is helpful in creating a window around the posterior aspect of the cystic duct to skeletonize the duct itself (Fig. 4). Alternatively, the tip of a hook-shaped cautery probe can be used to encircle and expose the duct. The cystic artery may be separated from the surrounding tissue by similar blunt dissection at this time or later, depending on its anatomic location. In the usual position, the cystic duct is dissected and divided first, as it is most anterior. If the cystic artery crosses anterior to the duct, dissection and division of the artery may be required prior to approaching the duct. Using the blunt concave blade of the spatula-tipped cautery as a Kittner dissector is often helpful during dissection of the cystic duct. Gentle irrigation is performed through the central lumen while the periductal structures are pushed away; this aids precise visualization.

Following initial dissection of the cystic duct, cholangiography may be performed. We perform this through the cystic duct, although other techniques may be employed. The dissecting forceps is used to squeeze gently the cystic duct in the direction of the gallbladder, thereby "milking"

Figure 5

cystic duct stones back into the gallbladder (Fig. 5). A clip applier placed through the epigastric sheath is used to affix a single clip to the junction of the cystic duct and the gallbladder. A scissors inserted through the axillary or midclavicular trocar is used to incise the anterolateral wall of the cystic duct, and the duct is milked again. A 4- or 5-F catheter is inserted through a gasketed hollow metal tube. The cholangiography catheter is inserted into the cystic duct and a clip is applied loosely to hold the catheter in place. If the introducer has grasping jaws it can be used to secure the

Figure 6

catheter into the duct (Fig. 6). If it is not possible to adequately expose the cystic duct using one of the accessory sheaths as a catheter introducer, a 4-F catheter may be inserted through a 14-gauge angiocatheter placed percutaneously. Two standard static radiographs are obtained following the injection of 3 or 4 mL and 10 mL of water-soluble contrast medium. Fluoroscopic cholangiography is the preferred method, as it allows dynamic real-time imaging.[26]

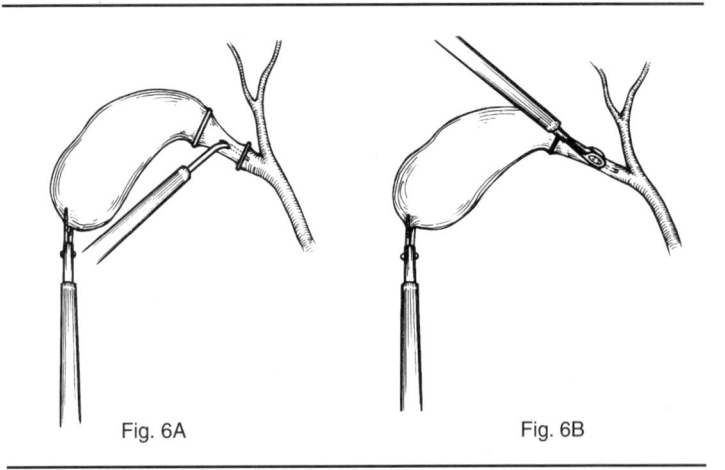

Fig. 6. Two techniques of cystic duct cholangiography after placement of a clip across the junction of the cystic duct and gallbladder. (A) Insertion of the catheter through a hollow tube into the cystic duct. A clip secures the catheter position. (B) Use of the cholangiography clamp. The catheter exits through the center of the clamp and the atraumatic jaws hold the catheter in place. (From Soper NJ.[15] Reproduced with permission.)

Figure 7

The film should be inspected to ascertain the size of the common bile duct, the location of the junction between the cystic duct and the common bile duct, the presence of intraluminal filling defects, the free flow of contrast medium into the duodenum, the anatomy of the proximal biliary tree, and the presence of any aberrant biliary radicles entering the gallbladder directly (Fig. 7).

After removal of the cholangiocatheter, the cystic duct is clipped doubly near its junction with the common bile duct and divided. The posterior jaw of the clip applier must be visualized prior to the application of each clip to avoid injury to the surrounding structures. Great care should be taken so that the common bile duct is not tented up into the clip. If the cystic duct is particularly large or friable, it may be preferable to replace one of the clips with a hand-tied or preformed suture.

Following this, attention is directed to the cystic artery. The assistant places the infundibulum of the gallbladder on tension and bluntly dissects the cystic artery from the surrounding tissue. The surgeon must ascertain that the structure is the cystic artery and not the right hepatic artery looping up onto the neck of the gallbladder, which is seen frequently. After an appropriate length of cystic artery has been separated from the surrounding tissue, it is doubly clipped proximally and distally, and divided sharply. Electrocautery should not be used for this division, as the current may be transmitted to the proximal clips, leading to necrosis

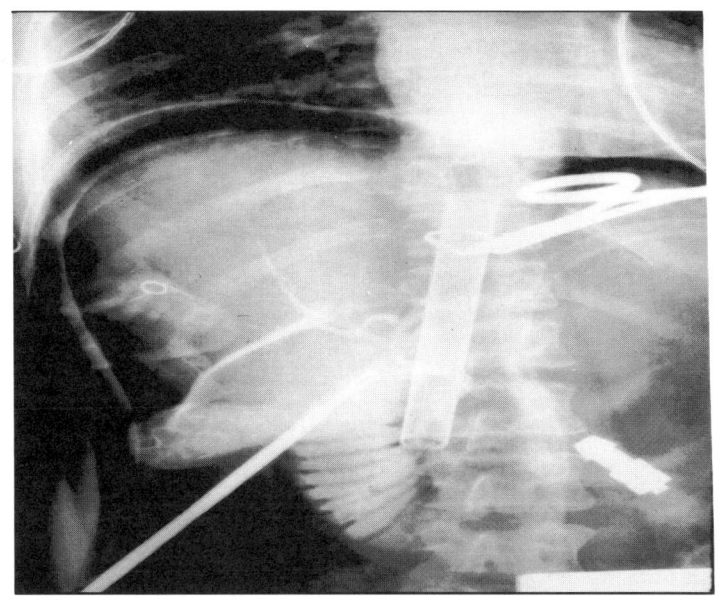

Fig. 7. Cholangiogram demonstrating contrast medium entering the gallbladder despite occlusion of the cystic duct, presumably due to an aberrant communication (duct of Luschka) between the liver and the gallbladder. (From Soper NJ, Dunnegan DL.[40] Reproduced with permission.)

and hemorrhage. A common error is to dissect and divide the anterior branch of the cystic artery, mistaking it for the main cystic artery. This may result in hemorrhage from the posterior branch during dissection of the gallbladder fossa.

The ligated stumps of the duct and cystic artery are then examined to ensure that there is no leakage of bile or blood, that the clips have been placed securely, and that they compress the entire lumen of the structures without impinging on adjacent tissue. No dissection is undertaken medial to the stumps; this prevents injury to structures in the porta hepatis. A suction-irrigation catheter is used to remove any debris or blood that may have accumulated during the dissection of the duct and artery. The heavy grasping forceps traversing the midclavicular trocar is repositioned on the proximal end of the gallbladder at Hartmann's pouch. The infundibulum is retracted superiorly and laterally and distracted anteriorly from its hepatic bed. The surgeon uses the dissecting forceps to thin out the tissue that tethers the neck of the gallbladder and ensure that there are no other sizable tubular structures traversing the space. Dissection of the hepatic fossa is then initiated using a thermal source to divide and coagulate small vessels and lymphatics. Occasionally a larger blood vessel or aberrant small bile duct will require placement of a clip for control.

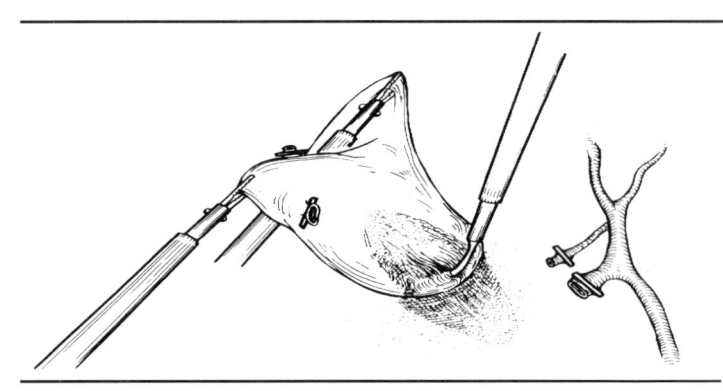

Fig. 8. Separation of the gallbladder from its bed by dissection with a blunt-tipped thermal energy probe. The neck of the gallbladder is placed on traction in a superior direction and then twisted to the left and right to place tension on the junction between the gallbladder and the hepatic fossa. (From Soper NJ.[15] Reproduced with permission.)

Once the appropriate plane has been identified, the separation of the gallbladder from its bed is performed by electrocautery or with laser-based instruments (Fig. 8). Appropriate traction and countertraction on the gallbladder facilitates the dissection tremendously. While the axillary forceps maintains cephalad traction on the fundus of the gallbladder, the midclavicular forceps pulls the neck of the gallbladder anterosuperiorly and then twists back and forth from medial to lateral to expose the right and left sides of the gallbladder, respectively. The jaws of the forceps on the fundus and neck should be distracted as widely as possible. With the tissue connecting the gallbladder to its fossa thus placed under tension, the surgeon uses an electrocautery spatula or hook in a gentle sweeping motion with low power (25 to 30 W) to coagulate and divide the tissue. Using the cautery probe it is also possible to perform blunt dissection, pushing the tissue to facilitate exposure of the proper plane. Occasionally hemorrhage from the liver bed or gallbladder obscures precise identification of the anatomy. Frequent irrigation through the port of the electrocautery instrument during this dissection clarifies visualization of the plane.

Alternatively, the dissection can be accomplished with a variety of laser tips, bipolar cautery, or other thermal devices. Lasers and electrocautery divide and coagulate blood vessels while removing the gallbladder from its bed. It is most effective to employ a sweeping or "painting" motion from left to right, creating a horizontal line of dissection. The generation of some smoke is unavoidable but generally does not obscure the view unless the liver substance is entered inadvertently. In such an instance a smoke evacuation system may be useful. Vaporized tissue fluid may fog the lens of the laparoscope. This is particularly problematic with edematous gallbladders and during dissection of the superior portion of the hepatic fossa. Usually the condensation clears within a few seconds but may require intermittent removal of the laparoscope to clean the lens with a dry sponge.

Dissection of the gallbladder fossa continues from the infundibulum to the fundus. The midclavicular grasping forceps is moved intermittently closer to the plane of dissection to allow maximal countertraction. The dissection proceeds until only a thin bridge of tissue remains to hold the gallbladder. At this point, prior to losing visualization of the operative field afforded by cephalad traction applied to the gallbladder, the hepatic fossa and porta hepatis are inspected again for hemostasis and bile leakage. Small bleeding points are coagulated with the electrocautery. The right upper quadrant is then irrigated liberally and aspirated dry. The final attachments of the gallbladder are lysed and the liver edge is examined once again for hemostasis. The assistant ensures that he or she has an adequate grasp on the gallbladder and pushes it onto the anterior surface of the right lobe of the liver. The position of the operating table is changed to return the patient to a full neutral supine position. This allows some of the irrigant that had been sequestered in the lower abdomen to return to the right upper quadrant and be aspirated.

Following cholecystectomy, the gallbladder must be removed from the abdominal cavity. This is done through the umbilicus because there are no muscle layers and only one fascial plane to traverse. Also, if the fascial opening needs to be enlarged to allow the removal of large or numerous stones, extension of the umbilical incision results in less postoperative pain than does enlargement of the subxiphoid entry site. The laparoscope is removed from the umbilical port and placed into the epigastric sheath. The pelvis and lower abdomen are inspected to ensure that there is no evidence of unappreciated injury to the bowel, bladder, or retroperitoneal blood vessels. The umbilical trocar insertion site is examined for hemorrhage. A large "claw" grasping forceps is introduced through the umbilical sheath and guided to the right upper quadrant. The assistant moves the neck of the gallbladder into the jaws of the grasper so that it is parallel to the axis of the forceps. The assistant then releases the gallbladder and its infundibulum is pulled up into the umbilical sheath. The forceps, sheath, and gallbladder neck are then retracted as a unit through the umbilical incision. The neck of the gallbladder is thus exposed on the anterior abdominal wall with the distended fundus remaining within the abdominal cavity (Fig. 9).

Figure 9

If the gallbladder is not distended with bile or stones it can be withdrawn with gentle traction. In most cases, Kelly

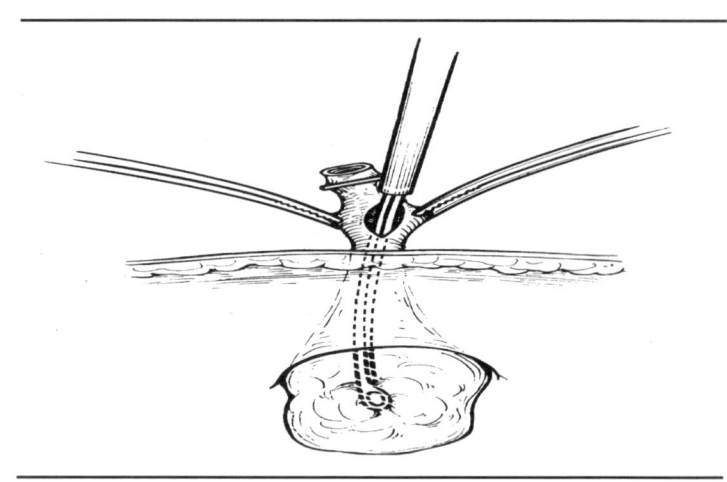

Fig. 9. Crushing or removal of gallstones contained within the fundus following delivery of the neck of the gallbladder through the umbilical incision. (From Soper NJ.[15] Reproduced with permission.)

clamps are placed on each side of the gallbladder neck and sponges are placed around the incision prior to opening the infundibulum. A suction catheter is introduced into the gallbladder to aspirate any bile and small stones. A stone forceps can be placed into the gallbladder to extract or crush calculi if necessary (Fig. 9). Occasionally the fascial incision must be extended to facilitate the removal of larger stones. After the gallbladder is extracted, the operator's finger is used to occlude the trocar site. If any question remains concerning hemostasis or contamination of the right upper quadrant, the umbilical trocar and sheath can be replaced under direct vision and the upper abdomen irrigated copiously and the fluid aspirated. Otherwise, the laparoscopic sheaths are opened to deflate the abdomen. Placing the patient in a slight Trendelenburg position may facilitate the escape of carbon dioxide trapped beneath the diaphragm. The sheaths are then removed.

Each incision is infiltrated with 0.5% bupivacaine to decrease postoperative discomfort, and irrigated with saline solution. The fascia of the umbilical incision is closed with one or two large absorbable sutures. The skin of the subxiphoid and umbilical incisions is closed with subcuticular absorbable sutures, and Steri-Strips are applied to each incision.

SPECIAL CONSIDERATIONS IN THE PERFORMANCE OF LAPAROSCOPIC CHOLECYSTECTOMY
Anatomic Hazards

The surgeon performing laparoscopic cholecystectomy must be aware of anatomic hazards that may lead to complications.

Avoiding complications: Common bile duct and cystic ducts

The common bile duct may be tented up due to the vigorous superolateral traction placed on the gallbladder, making it susceptible to injury during clip placement. Likewise, dissection in the region of the lateral wall of the common bile duct may cause bleeding from its nutrient vessels. Electrocautery must be avoided in this area, as subsequent devascularization and stricture may occur. Absent or extremely short cystic ducts may lead to two potential problems: the common bile duct may be mistaken for the cystic duct, and it may be extremely difficult to occlude the cystic duct with a clip if its length is insufficient. In these circumstances the surgeon may need to convert to an open cholecystectomy or leave a small portion of gallbladder infundibulum, which is closed with a laparoscopic suture.

Anomalous hepatic and cystic arteries

Aberrant bile ducts also may be present. If they are not recognized and ligated, direct communications between the biliary system and the gallbladder bed may lead to postoperative bile collections.[6] Aberrant origin of the right hepatic duct is common and must be ruled out in every case. Anomalous hepatic and cystic arteries may be present as well. In our experience the most common anomaly has been a right hepatic artery that loops up onto the infundibulum of the gallbladder. In such a case the cystic artery must be dissected up onto the gallbladder wall, clipped, and divided to allow the hepatic artery to retract away from the operative field. Finally, patients with a large left hepatic lobe may pose special problems. The epigastric trocar must be placed in an appropriate location so that instruments can enter the operative field from an angle at which they do not lacerate the left liver lobe, as occurred in one of our cases. If needed, an extra 5-mm port can be placed for insertion of a blunt probe to retract the left hepatic lobe during the operation.

Large left liver lobe

Conversion to Open Operation

Table 3

Surgeons performing laparoscopic cholecystectomy should not hesitate to convert to a traditional open procedure if the anatomy is unclear or complications arise (Table 3). It is better to "open one too many than to open one too few." Some complications requiring laparotomy are obvious, such as massive hemorrhage, bowel perforation, and major injury to the bile duct. An additional indication for open laparotomy is anatomy that cannot be delineated as a result of inflammation, adhesions, or anomalies. In general, if the gallbladder itself cannot be identified within 1 hour, the operation should be converted. This has happened to us on one occasion due to severe acute inflammation. Fistulas between the biliary system and bowel are not common,[27] but generally require laparotomy. Finally, the demonstration of potentially resectable carcinoma dictates open exploration.

Indications for open laparotomy

Table 3. Reasons to Convert to Open Cholecystectomy

Known or suspected injury to major blood vessel, viscus, or bile duct

Unclear anatomy

Unexpected pathology not amenable to laparoscopic management

Inability to remove common bile duct stone laparoscopically with little chance of subsequent endoscopic extraction (Billroth II anastomosis, duodenal diverticulum, previously failed ERCP)

Acute Cholecystitis

Acute cholecystitis may complicate the performance of laparoscopic cholecystectomy. Intervention during the early phase of the disorder reveals an inflamed, thick-walled, tensely distended organ. It may be necessary to decompress the gallbladder by aspiration with a large-gauge needle to gain purchase for the grasping forceps. As long as the inflammation is limited to the gallbladder it is usually technically feasible to perform laparoscopic cholecystectomy. However, if the inflammation extends to the porta hepatis, great care must be taken in proceeding with the operation. The normally thin, minimally adherent tissue that invests the cystic duct and artery is markedly thickened and edematous and may not be readily separable from these structures by the usual blunt dissection techniques. The duct wall may be edematous as well, making its external diameter similar to those of the gallbladder neck and common bile duct. If the anatomy is unclear a cholangiogram must be performed prior to clipping or dividing the tissue. If acute inflammation has been present for several days or weeks prior to surgery, the pericholecystic tissue planes may by obliterated by thick, woody tissue that is impossible to dissect bluntly. In such an instance, the surgeon may need to convert to open cholecystectomy if laparoscopic surgery is initiated during this subacute phase.

The ability to perform laparoscopic cholecystectomy should not influence the management of patients with acute cholecystitis.[28] Antibiotics and bowel rest are initiated upon admission to the hospital, and the operation is undertaken within 24 to 48 hours. There is no harm in inserting the laparoscope and assessing the right upper quadrant. The subcostal working ports are placed and the initial dissection is performed. If the anatomy is obliterated, a laparotomy is performed; if laparoscopic dissection is possible, the operation is completed. The decision to convert to an open operation is a matter of judgment based on the existing anatomy

Conversion to open operation is a matter of judgment

and the surgeon's experience. A number of authors have reported performing laparoscopic cholecystectomy in the face of acute inflammation.[29-31] Despite a greater incidence of conversion to open surgery, the operation may be completed safely in the majority of patients.

Intraoperative Gallbladder Perforation

Intraoperative spillage should not require conversion

Perforation of the gallbladder with leakage of bile or stones can be a distressing problem, but should not necessitate conversion to an open cholecystectomy. Perforation may occur secondary to traction applied by the grasping forceps or as a result of thermal injury during removal of the gallbladder from its bed. Almost one third of our patients have had some intraoperative spillage of bile and/or stones. However, patients with a bile leak did not experience an increased incidence of infection or prolongation of hospitalization or postoperative disability.[32] The only difference between those with and those without bile leakage was that surgery was approximately 10 minutes longer in patients with a gallbladder perforation, presumably as a result of the time spent cleaning up the operative field. When perforation does occur, the bile should be aspirated completely and irrigation used liberally. The stones should be retrieved and removed. Escaped stones composed primarily of cholesterol pose little threat of infection. However, pigment stones frequently harbor viable bacteria and may lead to subsequent infectious complications if allowed to remain in the peritoneal cavity.[33]

Cholangiography

As with traditional open cholecystectomy, intraoperative cholangiography can be performed during laparoscopic cholecystectomy routinely or on a selective basis.[26,34] There are many ardent advocates of both approaches and, just as with open cholecystectomy, this debate will probably remain unresolved. However, it is critical that the surgeon performing laparoscopic cholecystectomy have the capability to perform cholangiography when needed. There are several reasons for performing cholangiography selectively:

Capability for cholangiography is crucial

(1) Cholangiocatheter insertion is slightly more difficult and time-consuming than insertion with an open operative field; (2) catheter perforation or avulsion of the cystic duct may occur, injuring the common bile duct[35]; and (3) the incidence of false-positive findings on cholangiography may be even greater than the 3% to 9% seen with open cholecystectomy,[36] due to the associated hardware and longer dead space in the cholangiographic tubing. The indications for selective cholangiography are the same as those for open cholecystectomy. In addition, a dilated cystic duct measuring >4 mm or unclear anatomy necessitates cholangiography during laparo-

scopic cholecystectomy. Advocates of routine cholangiography during laparoscopic cholecystectomy state that roentgenologic delineation of the biliary anatomy is necessary to prevent major bile duct injury and to facilitate the detection and removal of ductal stones.[26,37-39]

Recently we reported a prospective randomized trial of static cholangiography during laparoscopic cholecystectomy.[40] In patients without perioperative indications for cholangiography, the technique added significant time and expense to the operation and did not influence outcome. Therefore, we feel that if only static cholangiography is available it need not be performed routinely for the safe performance of laparoscopic cholecystectomy. However, digital fluoroscopic equipment recently has become available for our use, and we now perform cholangiography routinely to train surgical residents in the technique and develop the technical skills that facilitate the laparoscopic management of choledocholithiasis.

Complications of Laparoscopic Cholecystectomy

Complications related to laparoscopy

Complications of laparoscopic cholecystectomy are due either to the laparoscopy or the cholecystectomy. Laparoscopic complications occur secondary to the carbon dioxide pneumoperitoneum or the instruments inserted through the abdominal wall. The complications of pneumoperitoneum (eg, gas embolism, vagal reaction, ventricular arrhythmias, hypercarbia with acidosis) have been discussed previously. Insertion of the initial trocar, especially when performed in a closed fashion, may injure the bowel, bladder, aorta, iliac artery, or vena cava, requiring open repair.[7] In contrast, if the small-bore Veress needle enters a viscus or blood vessel, the operation usually can be completed, and the patient monitored closely for signs of complications postoperatively. The laparoscopic trocars also may lacerate blood vessels in the abdominal wall. Prior to removing the trocars, they should be visualized from the peritoneal aspect by the laparoscope. If significant hemorrhage is seen, it can be controlled by placing a through-and-through bolstered suture on each side of the trocar insertion site.

Complications related to cholecystectomy

Complications related to removal of the gallbladder are similar to those related to traditional open cholecystectomy, and include hemorrhage, bile leak, and injury to a major bile duct. In early published reports, postoperative accumulations of bile not associated with a demonstrable biliary ductal injury seemed to occur more frequently with laparoscopic cholecystectomy than with traditional cholecystectomy.[41] This may have been a result of dissecting a plane further from the gallbladder surface with unrecognized damage to a superficial biliary radicle or a duct of Luschka.[42] The clips

Fig. 10A   Fig. 10B

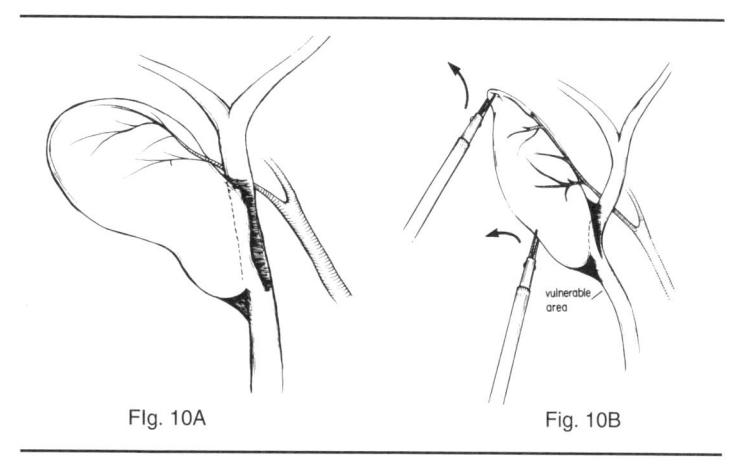

Fig. 10. (A) The "tethered infundibulum" obscuring the cystic duct. (B) With axial traction of the gallbladder, the common bile duct may be mistaken for the cystic duct and is therefore vulnerable to injury.

placed on the cystic duct stump may dislodge, leading to a postoperative bile leak. It may be possible to manage this complication by the percutaneous placement of drainage catheters with or without nasobiliary drains inserted endoscopically.

In the early experience of some authors[8,9] the reported incidence of major bile duct injuries was greater with laparoscopic cholecystectomy than with traditional open cholecystectomy. The accepted rate of bile duct injuries during standard cholecystectomy is 0% to 0.45%,[43] but this difference likely represents the learning curve rather than a permanent shortcoming of the technique.[8] The most frequent cause of bile duct injury during laparoscopic cholecystectomy is mistaking the common bile duct for the cystic duct. Because of the two-dimensional nature of laparoscopic imaging, traction applied to the gallbladder that causes the cystic duct to parallel the common bile duct can make a small-diameter common bile duct appear to be a continuation of the cystic duct. Alternatively, inflammation of the gallbladder neck can lead to adherence of the infundibulum to the common bile duct, obscuring a short cystic duct (Fig. 10). If the anatomy is not appreciated and cholangiography is not performed, the common bile duct will be excised with the gallbladder, leading to a high-level (grade 3 or 4) ductal injury. If a cholangiocatheter is inserted into the common bile duct and cholangiograms are obtained, contrast medium will flow into the duodenum but there will be no visualization of the proximal ducts (Fig. 11). Such a cholangiographic appearance should alert the surgeon to the likelihood of

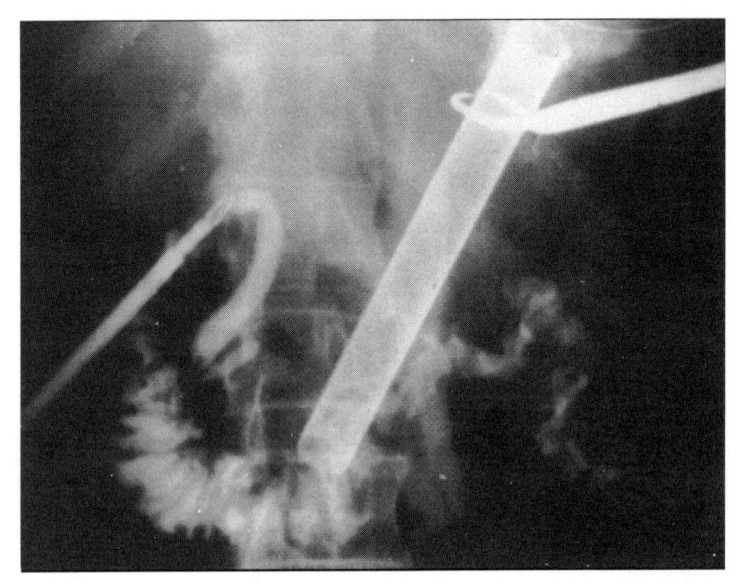

Fig. 11. Intraoperative cholangiogram demonstrating the absence of filling the proximal biliary tree. Laparotomy revealed intubation of the common bile duct just distal to the cystic duct insertion. (From Soper NJ.[15] Reproduced with permission.)

common bile duct cannulation. In this case, maneuvers to fill the proximal ducts (eg, administering morphine to cause spasm of the sphincter of Oddi, placing the patient in a head-down position) will not be successful, and the surgeon must convert to an open operation to delineate the anatomy and correct the problem. We have had one such bile duct injury caused by insertion of the cholangiocatheter; however, cholangiography did not cause the injury but rather prevented a catastrophic bile duct excision. The ductomy was treated simply by insertion of a T-tube with subsequent postoperative balloon dilatation. The patient has experienced no further sequelae.

Several technical points of the dissection that relate to common bile duct injury are worth reviewing: (1) The dissection should begin on the gallbladder and proceed toward the common bile duct rather than in the opposite direction. (2) Traction on the gallbladder infundibulum by the forceps introduced through the midclavicular ports should be applied posteriorly and laterally to expose Calot's triangle and position the cystic duct at right angles to the common bile duct. Excessive axial traction may cause tenting of the common bile duct and increase the likelihood of ductal dissection and injury. (3) Dissection should be carried out in Calot's triangle and the dorsal aspect of Calot's triangle by alternating lateral and medial traction on the gallbladder infundibulum. This maneuver will often serve to clarify the three-dimensional relationships of the cystic duct, hepatic duct, and common bile duct. The use of an angled (30° or 45°) telescope, which provides superior visualization of the common bile duct compared with the 0° scope, also may give an alternate view of Calot's triangle. (4) Identification of the cystic duct as it widens into the gallbladder must be achieved without exception. (5) Excessive dissection of the junction of the cystic duct and common bile duct is unnecessary and may lead to ischemic injury to the shoulder of the common bile duct. (6) Cholangiography must be performed if there is any uncertainty regarding the anatomy.[44] Injuries to the common bile duct usually mandate conversion to an open procedure with standard methods of repair or biliary reconstruction.[45]

POSTOPERATIVE CARE

Patients may be observed in the hospital or be discharged later the same day following laparoscopic cholecystectomy. We routinely keep patients overnight to monitor for immediate complications. It seems reasonable to perform laparoscopic cholecystectomy on an outpatient basis on responsible individuals who live with another person near a hospital, and patients without acute cholecystitis, urinary retention, or persistent nausea. Orders are written for antiemetics and analgesics as needed. Patients are allowed clear liquids in the immediate postoperative period and are advanced to a regular diet as tolerated. Nausea and shoulder pain due to diaphragmatic irritation may occur soon after surgery. No activity restrictions are placed on patients, whose functional status depends entirely upon the degree of abdominal tenderness, which usually subsides by the second or third postoperative day. Patients may return to work as soon as their abdominal discomfort becomes tolerable, but they are encouraged to do so within 1 week. We routinely evaluate patients in the office 1 month postoperatively; they also can be seen sooner should they have cause for concern.

RESULTS OF LAPAROSCOPIC CHOLECYSTECTOMY
Author's Personal Series

In mid-1989 a team of surgeons, including myself, at Washington University, St Louis, Missouri, first used the porcine model to develop the technique of laparoscopic cholecystectomy. We used monopolar electrocautery to dissect the gallbladder from its bed and were successful in extracting the gallbladder in eleven consecutive cases.[46] These results encouraged us to initiate a clinical series of laparoscopic cholecystectomies at Barnes Hospital at the Washington University Medical Center. A research protocol was submitted to the Human Studies Committee, and laparoscopic cholecystectomy was approved for clinical

Table 4. Compiled Results of Laparoscopic Cholecystectomy

Series	n	Converted to Open Laparotomy (%)	Mortality (%)	Major Complications (%)	Bile Duct Injury (%)
The Southern Surgeons Club[8] (1991)	1,518	4.7	0.07	1.5	0.5
Cuschieri, et al[12] (1991)	1,236	3.6	0.00	1.6	0.3
Soper, et al[10] (1992)	618	2.9	0.00	1.6	0.2
Spaw, et al[5] (1991)	500	1.8	0.00	1.0	0.0
Wolfe, et al[7] (1991)	381	3.0	0.90	3.4	0.0
Bailey, et al[11] (1991)	375	5.0	0.30	0.6	0.3
Graves, et al[13] (1991)	304	6.9	0.00	0.7	0.3
Peters, et al[6] (1991)	283	2.8	0.00	2.1	0.4
Schirmer, et al[9] (1991)	152	8.5	0.00	4.0	0.7

application.

Between November 1989 and November 1992 more than 1,500 laparoscopic cholecystectomies were performed at Washington University's affiliated hospitals; I was involved with more than 600 of these procedures. Our early results have been reported previously.[10] There have been no deaths within 30 days of surgery; major morbidity occurred in 1.6% of patients and minor morbidity occurred in 2.1% of patients (Table 4). The postoperative course of most patients has been uneventful, with 90% of patients being discharged from the hospital within 24 hours of surgery and only 11% requiring parenteral narcotics after leaving the recovery room. Similarly, the duration of disability has been minimal, with the average return to full activity occurring 8 days after surgery. These results compare favorably with those of traditional open cholecystectomy, following which most patients remain hospitalized for 3 to 5 days and do not return to work for 1 month.[16]

Other Reported Series

Our data reflect those of most series of laparoscopic cholecystectomies reported to date (Table 4). Death is rare following this procedure and usually is attributed to unrelated events. However, death has been reported as a result of injury to the bile duct or intestine.[7] The rate of conversion from the laparoscopic procedure to an open procedure ranges from

1.8% to 8.5% and tends to be greater early in the surgeon's experience with laparoscopy. Major complications, such as bile duct injury, have been relatively rare in the experience of surgeons who began performing laparoscopic cholecystectomy soon after its description.

Results of the National Institutes of Health Consensus Development Conference

Conclusions of 1992 Consensus Panel

Because of the prevalence of gallstones among the population of the United States, the cost borne by the health care system as a result of this disorder, and the rapid employment of laparoscopic cholecystectomy, the National Institute of Diabetes and Digestive and Kidney Diseases held a Consensus Development Conference titled, "Gallstones and Laparoscopic Cholecystectomy," from September 14 through September 16, 1992. The purpose of the conference was to evaluate and compare the data available on laparoscopic cholecystectomy and traditional surgical and nonsurgical approaches to the management of gallstones. The consensus panel, composed of surgeons, endoscopists, hepatologists, gastroenterologists, radiologists, epidemiologists, and representatives of the general public considered the scientific evidence presented by a number of experts in relevant fields. Several conclusions were reached: (1) Most asymptomatic patients with cholelithiasis should not be treated, but symptomatic patients should be treated promptly. (2) Laparoscopic cholecystectomy has become the treatment of choice for many patients, providing the advantages of decreased pain and disability and, potentially, substantially reduced cost. However, the outcome of laparoscopic cholecystectomy is influenced greatly by the training, experience, skill, and judgment of the surgeon performing the procedure. (3) Open cholecystectomy is a safe and effective operation for patients with symptomatic gallstone disease and remains the standard against which new treatments should be judged. Conversion from laparoscopy to open cholecystectomy should not be considered a complication of laparoscopic cholecystectomy. (4) Nonresective therapies for the management of gallstones have limited clinical applicability and require further development. (5) The management of common bile duct stones depends on the local availability of technical expertise. Valid treatment options include the preoperative, intraoperative, and postoperative identification and removal of stones. (6) Future research should focus on refining the techniques of laparoscopic cholecystectomy and laparoscopic common bile duct exploration to maximize safety and cost effectiveness. (7) Strict guidelines for training laparoscopic surgeons, determining their competence, and monitoring their quality should be developed and implemented promptly. (8) Safe, noninvasive,

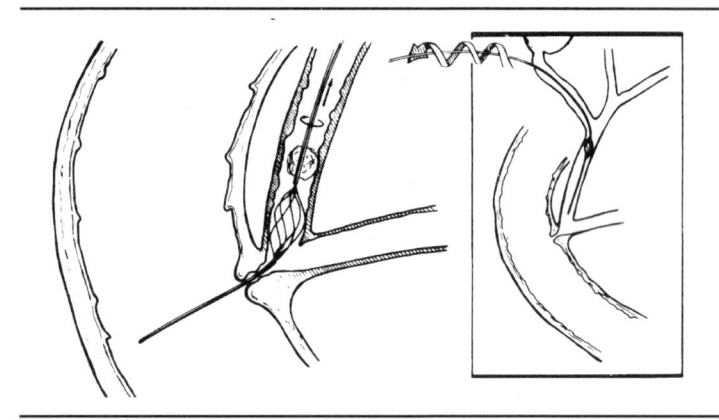

Fig. 12. Removal of a common bile duct stone. A six-wire helical stone basket is placed into the duct, and the duct is opened and "trolled" back, being rotated clockwise to entrap and remove the stone. (From Hunter JG, Soper NJ.[48] Reproduced with permission.)

Controversies in management

cost-effective strategies to prevent gallstones should be sought actively.

MANAGEMENT OF COMMON BILE DUCT STONES

Common bile duct stones may be present in up to 15% of patients with cholelithiasis.[47,48] Because laparoscopic techniques for extracting common bile duct stones are currently under development, the management of choledocholithiasis during laparoscopic cholecystectomy is controversial. These stones may be discovered preoperatively, intraoperatively, or postoperatively. When they are discovered preoperatively, the surgeon has a number of options. The most conservative mode of treatment is traditional open cholecystectomy with common bile duct exploration. However, this increases morbidity and mortality over that associated with cholecystectomy alone,[49] and subjects patients to a longer hospital stay and the presence of a T-tube in the common bile duct. The other therapeutic alternatives are endoscopic retrograde cholangiopancreatography (ERCP) with sphincterotomy and stone extraction, leaving the gallbladder in situ; preoperative ERCP/sphincterotomy with subsequent laparoscopic cholecystectomy; and laparoscopic cholecystectomy with attempted translaparoscopic extraction of the common bile duct stones and open choledochotomy or postoperative ERCP/sphincterotomy, if necessary.

Opinions differ on the adequacy of sphincterotomy and the extraction of common bile duct calculi in patients whose gallbladders contain stones.[50] Although the need for subsequent cholecystectomy has been relatively uncommon in large series of patients thus treated, this therapy seems less than ideal for patients who are medically fit to undergo general anesthesia. Because of the vagaries of the intraoperative extraction of common bile duct stones using laparoscopic techniques, many surgeons have opted for preoperative ERCP with stone extraction followed by laparoscopic cholecystectomy in patients with cholelithiasis and suspected common bile duct stones. We followed this policy initially, demonstrating and removing common duct stones successfully in >50% of selected patients undergoing preoperative ERCP, with low morbidity.[51] Advantages of this approach *in the presence of an experienced endoscopist* include minimization of the operative time for the subsequent laparoscopic procedure, low morbidity (<10%), highly effective management of choledocholithiasis (>90% success rate), preoperative identification of those few patients not amenable to postoperative endoscopic management of retained duct stones, and maintenance of a minimally invasive approach.[52] Disadvantages of preoperative ERCP include the addition of a potentially dangerous procedure that is unnecessary in up to 80% of patients,[8] and the uncertain long-term effects of sphincterotomy.[50,52] Preoperative ERCP clearly is indicated in individuals with cholangitis, severe pancreatitis, or deep jaundice, as other conditions requiring additional intervention may be discovered in up to 40% of patients.[53,54]

Pros and cons of preoperative ERCP

Patients in whom stones in the common bile duct are discovered on intraoperative cholangiography pose a dilemma. The conservative approach would be to convert the operation to a standard open cholecystectomy and common bile duct exploration. For the surgeon inexperienced in the laparoscopic treatment of choledocholithiasis, this approach may be reasonable in patients with large, completely obstructing stones in whom a subsequent failed ERCP would carry potentially grave consequences, or in patients in whom preoperative ERCP has not been technically possible. Alternatively, patients with small nonobstructing stones may undergo completion of the cholecystectomy and subsequent ERCP postoperatively should symptoms arise. Finally, stones within the common bile dust usually can be removed translaparoscopically. Using fluoroscopic guidance, a helical stone basket may be passed through the cystic duct and into the common bile duct. The stone is then extracted by a technique similar to the T-tube extraction of retained common bile duct stones (Fig. 12).[55] Another approach is to dilate the cystic duct and pass through a small flexible ureteroscope (<10 F) into the common bile duct.[56-58] Under direct vision, the stones can be extracted using a four-wire Segura stone basket placed through the biopsy channel of the endoscope (Fig. 13) or fragmented using intracorporeal lithotripsy probes or stone lasers. However, this technique is limited by a relative inability to visualize the proximal biliary system. Yet, we

Figure 12

Figure 13

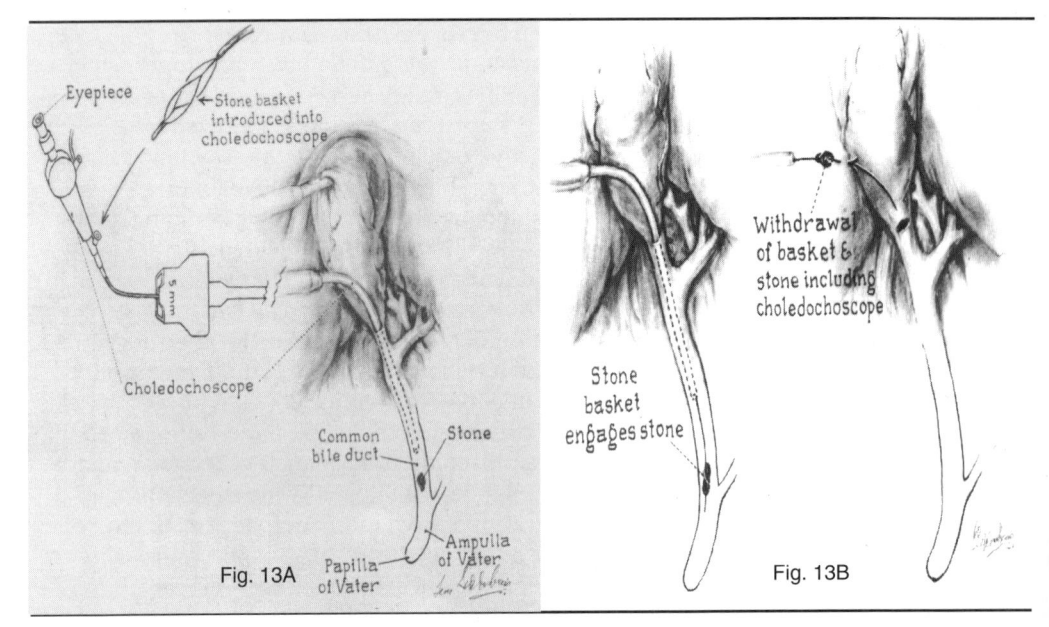

Fig. 13. (A) Insertion of a choledochoscope through the cystic duct into the common bile duct with (B) removal of stones under direct vision. (From Zucker K, Bailey R, in Zucker K [ed]. *Surgical Laparoscopy Update*, St Louis, Mo, Quality Medical Publishing Inc, 1993. Reproduced with permission.)

have extracted bile duct stones successfully in a number of patients with this technique (Fig. 14). These patients are discharged on the first postoperative day and return to full activity within 1 week without being subjected to a second procedure or the presence of a T-tube.

Experience with these trans-cystic duct approaches to choledocholithiasis is increasing, and early results have been encouraging (Table 5). Currently this approach is dependent upon adequate technology and requires experience in safely accessing the cystic duct; the risk of injuring the proximal cystic or bile duct is unknown. Due to the cystic duct's usual angle of entry into the common bile duct it is difficult to manage stones found in the hepatic ducts. In the future many devices undoubtedly will be designed to simplify the laparoscopic management of common bile duct stones.

Experience with laparoscopic choledochotomy, stone extraction, and suture closure with a T-tube is limited.[58,59] This approach allows complete visualization of the biliary system but requires advanced suturing skills. Also, postoperative recuperation may mimic that of open choledochotomy rather than laparoscopic cholecystectomy.[58] Other novel approaches include antegrade sphincterotomy using a probe passed from above, through the cystic duct. Ductal stones that cannot be removed laparoscopically require open choledochotomy or postoperative ERCP. The precise role of each of these techniques for managing choledocholithiasis depends on local expertise and the patient's wishes.

Some patients are discovered to have retained common bile duct stones that were not detected during the perioperative period. As with patients in whom retained stones are discovered after standard open cholecystectomy, the initial approach here is endoscopic sphincterotomy with stone extraction or stone extraction using a percutaneous radiologic approach. The need to treat patients with small asymptomatic stones during the postoperative period is unclear. We observed one such patient who developed symptoms 18 months postoperatively, and was treated successfully with endoscopy. Of course, a retained stone that cannot be removed endoscopically or percutaneously in a symptomatic patient may necessitate open common bile duct exploration.

CONCLUSION

Laparoscopy has rapidly become the new gold standard for the management of gallstones in patients throughout the world. Most cases of symptomatic gallstones can be treated laparoscopically. Occasionally, anatomic or physiologic considerations will preclude the laparoscopic approach, but

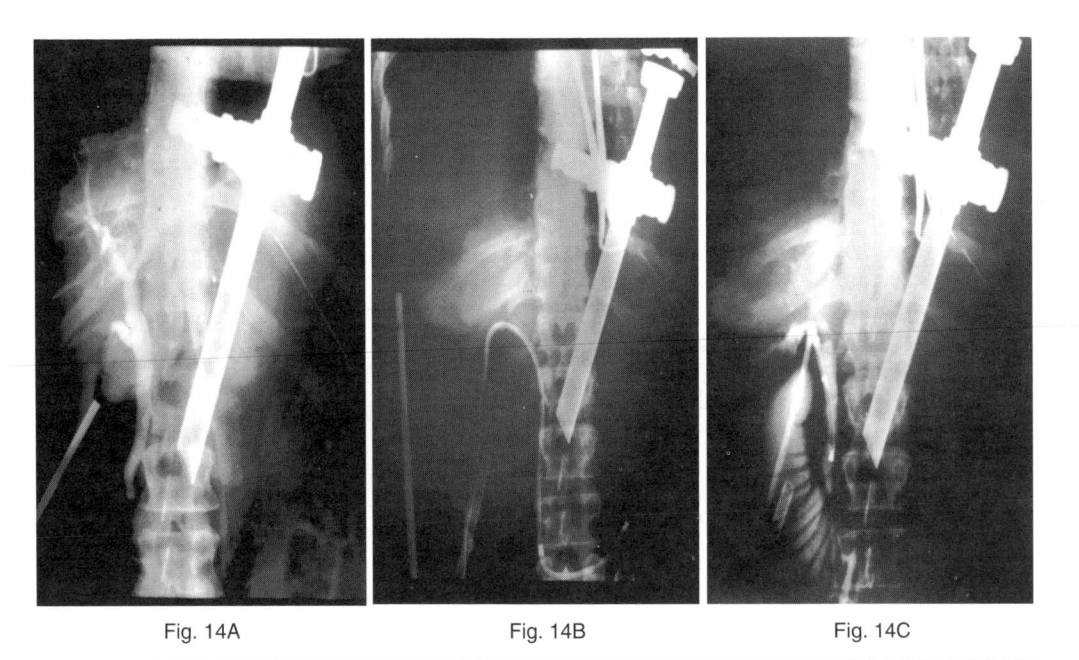

Fig. 14A   Fig. 14B   Fig. 14C

Fig. 14. Obstruction of the common bile duct stone managed by translaparoscopic extraction. (A) Initial cystic duct cholangiogram showing a meniscus filling defect of the distal common bile duct with an absence of flow into the duodenum. (B) A 9-F ureteroscope was placed through the cystic duct and the stone was extracted. The ureteroscope was then advanced into the duodenum, as shown. (C) The ureteroscope was next withdrawn into the common bile duct. A completion cholangiogram obtained through the scope demonstrates the absence of the stone and free flow of contrast medium into the duodenum. (From Smith PC, et al.[56] Reproduced with permission.)

Table 5. Management of Choledocholithiasis

Technique	Success (%)	Postoperative Stay (d)	RTW (d)
Trans-cystic duct extraction	75-93	1-2	7-10
Laparoscopic CBDE	85-100	4-7	14-30
Open CBDE	90-100	5-10	20-42
ERCP/sphincterotomy	85-95	2-3	7-14

RTW = Interval to return to work, CBDE = Common bile duct exploration, ERCP = Endoscopic retrograde cholangiopancreatography.

laparoscopy may be converted to an open operation. Such a decision reflects sound surgical judgment and should not be considered a complication. The optimal management of choledocholithiasis in the era of laparoscopic cholecystectomy remains to be determined by careful prospective studies. However, early results suggest that most patients may benefit greatly from the application of laparoscopic techniques to remove gallstones from the common bile duct, thereby preserving the minimally invasive approach and curing the patient with a single procedure. Undoubtedly, technologic developments in the next few years will simplify the laparoscopic approach to biliary disorders.

References
1. Mühe E. *Lang Arch Chir* 1986;369:804.
2. DuBois F, et al. *Ann Surg* 1990;211:60-62.
3. Perissat J, et al. *Surg Endosc* 1990;4:1-5.
4. Reddick EJ, Olsen DO. *Surg Endosc* 1989;3:131-133.
5. Spaw NJ, et al. *Surg Laparosc Endosc* 1992;127:917-921.
6. Peters JH, et al. *Surgery* 1991;110:769-778.
7. Wolfe BM, et al. *Arch Surg* 1991;126:1192-1196.
8. The Southern Surgeons Club. *N Engl J Med* 1991;324:1073-1078.
9. Schirmer BD, et al. *Ann Surg* 1991;213:665-676.
10. Soper NJ, et al. *Arch Surg* 1992;127:917-921.
11. Bailey RW, et al. *Ann Surg* 1991;214:531-540.
12. Cuschieri A, et al. *Am J Surg* 1991;161:385-387.
13. Graves HA, et al. *Ann Surg* 1991;213:655-662.
14. Goldsmith MF. *JAMA* 1990;264:2723.
15. Soper NJ. *Curr Probl Surg* 1991;28:585-655.
16. Soper NJ, et al. *Surg Gynecol Obstet* 1992;174:114-118.
17. Anderson ER, Hunter JG. *Surg Laparosc Endosc* 1991;1:82-84.
18. Fisher KS, et al. *Surg Laparosc Endosc* 1991;1:77-81.
19. Gracie WA, Ransohoff DF. *N Engl J Med* 1982;307:798-800.
20. Ransohoff DF, et al. *Ann Intern Med* 1983;99:199-204.
21. Soper NJ, et al. *Surg Endosc* 1992;6:115-117.
22. Stoelting RK, Miller RD, in *Basics of Anesthesia*. New York, NY, Churchill Livingstone, 1989, pp 211-227.

23. Gravenstein JS, et al, in *Capnography in Clinical Practice*. Boston, Mass, Butterworth Publishers, 1989, pp 3-10.
24. Kitano S, et al. *Surg Endosc* 1991;6:197-198.
25. Graff TD, et al. *Am J Obstet Gynecol* 1959;78;259-265.
26. Bruhn EW, et al. *Surg Endosc* 1991;5:111-115.
27. Remine WH. *Adv Surg* 1973;7:69-75.
28. Hermann RE. *Surg Clin North Am* 1990;70:1263-1275.
29. Cooperman AM. *J Laparosc Endosc Surg* 1990;1:37-40.
30. Reddick EJ, et al. *Am J Surg* 1991;161:377-381.
31. Unger SW, et al. *Surg Laparosc Endosc* 1991;1:14-16.
32. Soper NJ, Dunnegan DL. *Surg Laparosc Endosc* 1991;1:156-161.
33. Stuart L, et al. *Ann Surg* 1987;206:242-249.
34. Gregg RO. *Am J Surg* 1988;155:540-544.
35. White TT, Hart MJ. *Am J Surg* 1985;149:640-643.
36. Del Santo P, et al. *Surgery* 1985;98:7-11.
37. Berci G, et al. *Am J Surg* 1991;161:355-360.
38. Blattner ME, et al. *Arch Surg* 1991;126;646-649.
39. Phillips EH, et al. *Am Surg* 1990;56:792-795.
40. Soper NJ, Dunnegan DL. *World J Surg* 1992;16:1133-1140.
41. Peters JH, et al. *Ann Surg* 1991;213:3-12.
42. Luschka H. *Die Anatomie das Menschlichen Bauches*. Tubingen, H. Lauppschen, Bushhandlung 1863;255.
43. Gilliland TM, Traverso LW. *Surg Gynecol Obstet* 1990;170:39-44.
44. Way LW. *Ann Surg* 1992;215:195.
45. Pitt HA, et al. *Ann Surg* 1989;210:417-425.
46. Soper NJ, et al. *Surg Laparosc Endosc* 1991;1:17-22.
47. Mullen JL, et al. *Surg Gynecol Obstet* 1971;133:774-779.
48. Hunter JG, Soper NJ. *Surg Clin North Am* 1992;72:1077-1098.
49. Frazee RC, van Heerden JA. *Surg Gynecol Obstet* 1989;168:513-516.
50. Tanaka M, et al. *Am J Surg* 1987;154:505-509.
51. Aliperti G, et al. *Ann Intern Med* 1991;115:783-785.
52. Cotton PB, et al. *Gastrointest Endosc* 1991;37:383-393.
53. Gaisford WD. *Am J Surg* 1976;132:699-702.
54. Kullman E, et al. *Acta Chir Scand* 1984;150:657-663.
55. Hunter JG. *Am J Surg* 1992;163:53-58.
56. Smith PC, et al. *Surgery* 1992;111:230-233.
57. Petelin JB. *Surg Laparosc Endosc* 1991;1:33-41.
58. Phillips EH, et al. *World J Surg*, in press.
59. Stoker ME, et al. *J Laparosc Endosc Surg* 1991;1:287-293.

Index

Page numbers in **boldface** type refer to pages on which tables or figures appear; those followed by an *italic t* or *f* denote tables or figures, respectively.

Abscess
  appendiceal
    antibiotics (intravenous), 30
    initial appendectomy, 30
    interval appendectomy, 30
    operative drainage, 30
    percutaneous drainage, 30
Anesthesia
  laparoscopic cholecystectomy
    general inhalation, 45
    monitoring, 45
    regional anesthesia, 45
    thoracic epidural anesthesia, 45
Antibiotics
  acute cholecystitis, 60
  appendicitis
    appendiceal abscess, 30
    in uncomplicated, 30
Appendectomy
  laparoscopic
    efficacy vs open, 30
    history, 29
    incidental, 33
    indications, 29, 30
    interval appendectomy, 30
    method, 30–32
    results, 32–33
Appendicitis
  diagnosis
    clinical, 29
    laparoscopic, 29, 30

Bowel resection
  segmental colon, 21–29
  small bowel, 35

Cautery
  electrocautery
    in laparoscopic cholecystectomy,
      52, 53, 56, 57
    safety measures, 42
  laser cautery
    eye safety, 42
    laparoscopic cholecystectomy, 56
Cholangiography
  in laparoscopic cholecystectomy,
    53–54, **54***f*
    cholangiogram, **55***f*
    injury by cholangiocatheter
      of common bile duct, 63–64, **64***f*
    routine vs selective intraoperative
      cholangiography, 62
Cholecystitis
  acute, 60–61

    as complicating factor, 60–61
    management of patients, 60
Choledocholithiasis
  management, **72***t*
  stones discovered on intraoperative
    cholangiography, 69–71
    indications for completion of
      laparoscopic cholecystectomy, 69
    indications for conversion
      to open cholecystectomy, 68
    laparoscopic choledochotomy, 70
    removal of common bile duct stones,
      68–71, **68***f*, **70***f*, **71***f*
  stones discovered preoperatively, 68–69
    laparoscopic cholecystectomy with
      translaparoscopic extraction, 68–69
    open choledochotomy or
      postoperative ERCP
      sphincterotomy, 68
    sphincterotomy and stone
      extraction, 68
Choledochoscope, 43, **71***f*
Cholelithiasis
  diagnosis, 40–41
Clip appliers
  in laparoscopic cholecystectomy
  types and advantages, 43
Colonoscope
  specimen removal, 20
Colonoscopy
  segmental colon resection for
    intraoperative localization
    of lesion, 22, 25
Common bile duct stones,
  see *Choledocholithiasis*
Conversion to open surgery
  indications
    appendectomy, 30
    cholecystectomy, 59–60, **60***t*
    choledocholithiasis, 68–71
    intraoperative perforation, 61
    laparoscopic colectomies, 27

Endoscopic retrograde
  cholangiopancreatography (ERCP), 68
  advantages and disadvantages
    of preoperative ERCP, 68–69
  indications of preoperative ERCP, 69

Gallbladder
  cholecystectomy, 48–58

Hemostasis
  laparoscopic cholecystectomy, 42

laparoscopic colon resection, 23
Hernia repair
  anatomy of inguinal area
    muscles, tendons, ligaments, 2-4, **2f**, **3f**, **4f**
    nerve supply, 3
  complications, 16, **16t**
  herniorrhaphy glossary, **5t**
  history, 1–2
  inguinal hernias
    direct, 4–5, **7f**
    femoral, 4–5
    indirect, 4, **7f**
  results, **12t**, 13–16, **13t**
  selected anatomic features
    Cooper's ligament, **3f**, **4f**
    cremaster muscle, **2f**
    epigastric vessels, **4f**
    femoral artery, **2f**
    femoral sheath, **3f**
    femoral vein, **2f**
    iliac artery and vein, **4f**
    iliopectineal arch, **3f**
    iliopsoas muscle, **3f**
    iliopubic tract, **3f**, **4f**
    inguinal ligament, **2f**, **3f**
    internal abdominal oblique muscle, **2f**, **3f**
    internal abdominal ring, **3f**
    lacunal ligament, **2f**
    pubic ramus, **3f**
    public tubercle, **2f**, **4f**
    rectus muscle, **4f**
    superior iliac spine, **3f**
    vas deferens, **4f**
  techniques, 9–13
    laparoscopic approaches
      preperitoneal, 11–13
      transperitoneal, 9–11, **11f**
    standard approaches
      anatomic, 5
      anterior, 5
      Bassini, 5–6
      Halsted, 5–6
      intra-abdominal, 5
      McVay, 5–6
      nonanatomic, 5
      Shouldice, 6–7, **6f**

Instrument sets for laparoscopic cholecystectomy, 42

Laparoscopic appendectomy
  in children
    not indicated in those below 8 to 10 years of age, 30
    indicated in teenagers and adults, 30
  incidental, 33
  indications, 29–30
  interval appendectomy, 30
  methods, 30–32, **31f**, **32f**
  results, 32–33

"Laparoscopic-assisted resection"
  a more appropriate term, 20
Laparoscopic benefits
  appendectomy 31–33
  appendicitis diagnosis, 30
  intestinal surgery, 35
Laparoscopic cholecystectomy
  advantages, **39t**
  anatomic hazards, 58–59
  anesthesia, 44–45
  choledocholithiasis, 68–72
  comparison with other cholelithiasis therapies, **39t**
  complications, 62–65
    bile duct injuries, 62
    common bile duct mistaken for cystic duct, 62–64, **64f**
    initial trocar, 62
    other laparoscopic trocars, 62
    pneumoperitoneum, 48, 62
    removal of gallbladder, 62
    technical points of dissection related to common bile duct, 64-65
    "tethered infundibulum" obscures cystic duct, 62–64, **64f**
  contraindications, **40t**
  disadvantages, 39–40, **39t**
  equipment, 41–44
    balloon dilators, 44
    baskets for stone extraction, 43
    choledochoscopes, 43
    guide wires, 43
    insufflators, 41
    laparoscopes, 41–42
    laparoscopic cholecystectomy instrument sets, 42
    laparoscopic clip appliers, 43
    laparoscopic needle holders, 42
    probes for cautery, 42–43
    standard cholecystectomy set, 43
    trocars and sheaths, 42
    video camera, 42
    xenon light source, 41
  intraoperative gallbladder perforation, 61
  operating room organization, 43–44, **43f**
  pneumoperitoneum, 45–49
  postoperative care, 65
  recent history, 38
  results, 65–68
    author's personal series, 65–66, **66t**
    other series, 66–67, **66t**
    NIH Consensus Development Conference (1992): conclusions of Consensus Panel, 67–68
  techniques, 49–58
    Calot's triangle and reverse (dorsal aspect) for orientation, 51–53, **51f**
    completion of cholecystectomy, 57
    cystic duct cholangiography, 53–54, **54f**, **55f**

deflation of abdomen, 58
diagnosis and removal of cystic duct
 stones by "milking," 52–53, **52f**
insertion of initial laparoscopic
 sheath, **47f, 50f**
removal of gallbladder from
 abdominal cavity, 57–58, **58f**
removal of gallstones contained in
 fundus following delivery of neck
 through umbilical incision, **58f**
separation of gallbladder from its
 bed, 54–56, **56f**
Laparoscopic colon procedures
(other than resection)
 indications, 33–35, **34t**
 procedures, 33–35, **34t**
Laparoscopic colon resection
 indications, 20–21, **21t**
 method, 21–28, **22f, 23t, 24f, 28f**
 results, 26–28
Laparoscopic intestinal surgery
 appendectomy, 29–33
 colon resection, 20–29
 colostomy, 33–34, **34t**
 diverting colostomy, 33–34, **34t**
 diverting iliostomy, 33–34, **34t**
 gastrojejunostomy, 20
 Ripstein procedure, **34t**
 small bowel resection, 20

Mesh (prosthesis)
 hernia repair, 10–12

Operating room organization
 for laparoscopic biliary surgery, **43f**
Operating team
 for laparoscopic cholecystectomy,
  43, **43f**
 for laparoscopic segmental
  colon resection 21–22

Pneumoperitoneum
 laparoscopic appendectomy, 31
 laparoscopic cholecystectomy
  carbon dioxide, advantages
   and disadvantages, 45
  complications, 48, 62
  effects of carbon dioxide on fetus, 41
  establishment of, closed technique,
   46–48
  establishment of, open technique,
   45, 48–49
 laparoscopic hernia repair, 9
Proctoscopy
 intraoperative, 34

Sigmoid colectomy
 economics of, 27
 laparoscopic procedure, 27–28, **28f**
Sigmoidoscopy
 intraoperative, 34

Society of Colon and Rectal Surgery
 Registry, 29
Staplers
 appendectomy, 31–32
 colostomy, 34
 EEA-type circular, 28
 GIA-type
  extracorporeal intestinal
   anastomosis, **24f**
  intracorporeal intestinal
   anastomosis, 25
 ileostomy, 34
 Meckel's diverticulum, 35
 rectosigmoid resection, 26, 28
 right colon resection, 24
 segmental colon resection, 25
 TA-type, 34
Surgical specimens
 laparoscopic segmental colon
  resection, 24–25, **24f**, 27

Transillumination
 colon resection, 24–25, **24f**
Trendelenburg position
 indications in rectosigmoid resection, 26
 indications in segmental
  colon resection, 22
 in laparoscopic cholecystectomy, 49, 58
 pneumoperitoneum,
  closed technique, 46
Trocars
 disposable trocar/sheath assemblies, 41
 Hasson, 31
 hernia repair, 9
 laparoscopic appendectomy, 31
 laparoscopic cholecystectomy, 41

Ultrasound
 cholelithiasis diagnosis, 39

Vessel loops
 colon resection, 24

Xenon light source
 laparoscopic cholecystectomy, 41

NEW DATA

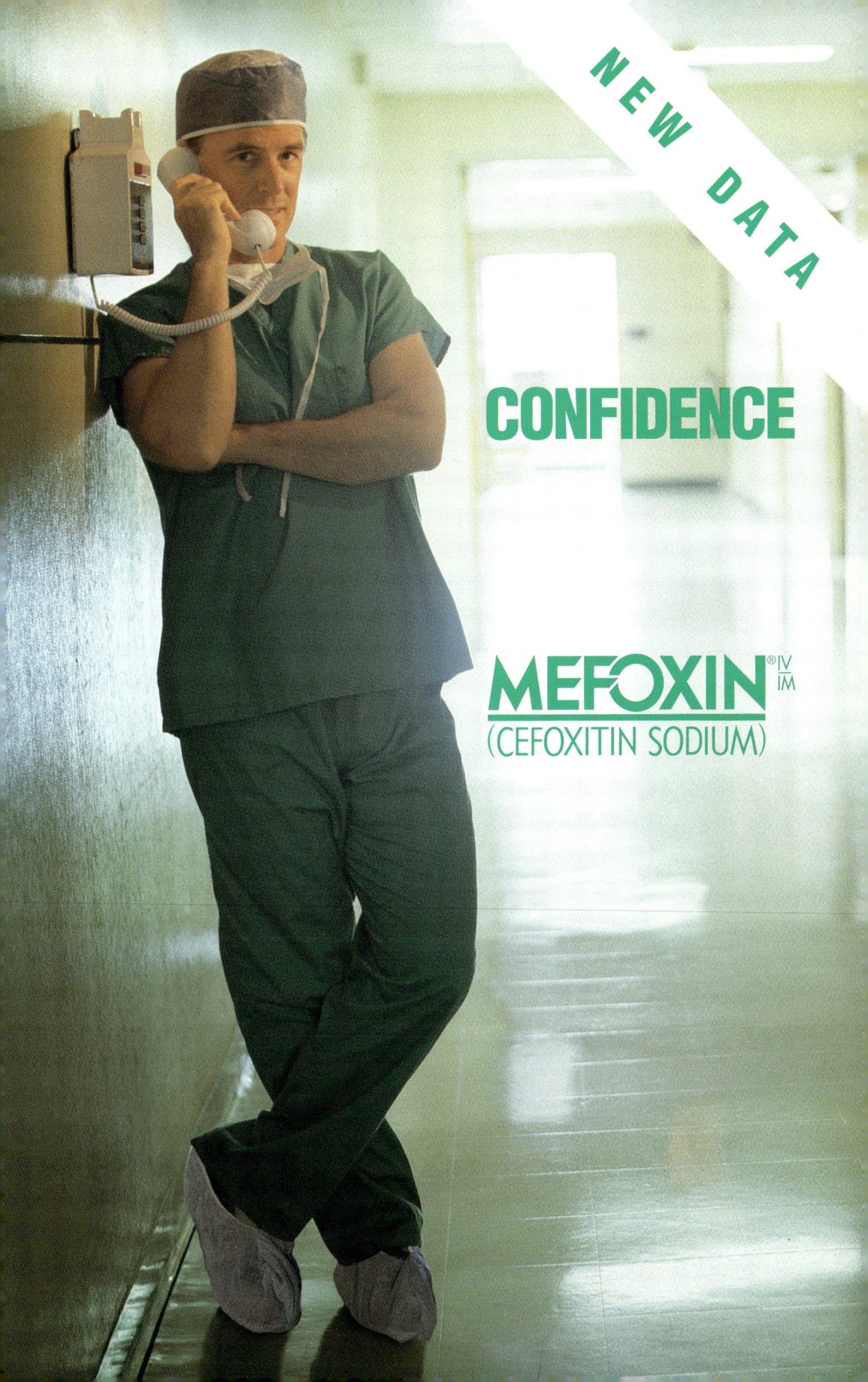

CONFIDENCE

MEFOXIN® IV/IM
(CEFOXITIN SODIUM)

In a recent study of patients
with acute colonic diverticulitis at five medical centers[1]

AS EFFECTIVE AS COMBINATION THERAPY

MEFOXIN® (Cefoxitin Sodium)	Cured* 90%
Gentamicin-Clindamycin	Cured 86%

0 — 50 — 100

The difference in cure rates was not statistically significant.

MEFOXIN			Gentamicin-Clindamycin	
Number of patients	30		Number of patients	21
Number cured	27*(90%)		Number cured	18 (86%)
Number failed	3 (10%)		Number failed	3 (14%)

* Includes 6 patients considered cured of acute diverticulitis who had elective one-step operations without septic complications. All 6 had had previous hospitalizations for acute diverticulitis.

Simpler to administer and potentially more cost-effective than gentamicin-clindamycin[1]

- Single-agent simplicity of administration
- No need for serum level determinations
- 15% cost savings demonstrated in the one center which performed a cost analysis**

MEFOXIN is not active *in vitro* against most strains of *Pseudomonas aeruginosa* and enterococci (e.g., *Streptococcus faecalis*) and many strains of *Enterobacter cloacae*. Methicillin-resistant staphylococci are almost uniformly resistant to MEFOXIN.

MEFOXIN is contraindicated in patients who have shown hypersensitivity to cefoxitin and the cephalosporin group of antibiotics.

Pseudomembranous colitis, from mild to life-threatening in severity, has been reported with virtually all antibiotics (including cephalosporins); therefore, it is important to consider its diagnosis when diarrhea develops in association with antibiotic use.

** Only one center studied comparative costs. The 15% cost savings at this center was attributed to differences in drug acquisition and administration costs (i.e., serum level assays and staff costs).
1. Kellum, J.M. et al., *Clin. Ther.*, 1992

In a study by Goldstein and Citron[2]

ANAEROBES: OVERALL *IN VITRO*[***] COVERAGE OF THE *B. fragilis* GROUP BETTER THAN CEFOTAN[††]

In vitro susceptibilities of isolates from two community hospitals at a 32-mcg/mL breakpoint (n=215)[2]

	B. fragilis	B. thetaiota-omicron	B. distasonis	B. vulgatus	B. ovatus
MEFOXIN	**97%**	**92%**	**69%**	**93%**	**82%**
Cefotan	93%	24%	16%	93%	12%

NOTE: Based on the 1993 *Physicians' Desk Reference*®, Cefotan is usually active *in vitro* and in clinical infections against a number of organisms, including *Bacteroides* species (excluding *B. distasonis*, *B. ovatus*, and *B. thetaiotaomicron*).

In a study by Gill et al.[3]

AEROBES: *IN VITRO*[***] COVERAGE OF *E. coli* AND *Klebsiella* spp. BETTER THAN ($p \leq 0.0001$)[†††] AMPICILLIN/SULBACTAM

In vitro susceptibilities at a concentration of 8 mcg/mL[3]	*E. coli* (n=293)	*Klebsiella* spp. (n=160)
MEFOXIN	**97%**	**98%**
Ampicillin/Sulbactam	75%	83%

A bacterial isolate may be considered susceptible if the MIC value for cefoxitin is not more than 16 mcg/mL. Organisms are considered resistant to cefoxitin if the MIC is greater than 32 mcg/mL.
The susceptibility breakpoint for Unasyn® (Pfizer Inc.) is 8 mcg/mL, as stated in the 1993 *Physicians' Desk Reference*®.

[***] *In vitro* activity does not necessarily imply *in vivo* efficacy.
[††] registered trademark of Imperial Chemical Industries for cefotetan disodium
[†††] Statistical significance calculated postpublication for both species using McNemar's test. (Data available upon request from Professional Services, Merck & Co., Inc., West Point, PA 19486. Please request information package #DA-FOX 1.)

BALANCED COVERAGE[†] WITH

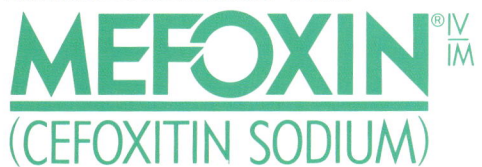

MEFOXIN® IV/IM
(CEFOXITIN SODIUM)

[†] Denotes *in vitro* activity against indicated aerobes and anaerobes. This does not necessarily imply *in vivo* efficacy.

2. Goldstein, E.J.C. and Citron, D.M., *J. Clin. Microbiol.*, 1988
3. Gill, C.J. et al., *Clin. Ther.*, 1991

A Preferred Choice...
FOR SIGNIFICANT MEDICAL REASONS

- Clinical experience in over 18 million patients*
- Balanced coverage† of many important aerobes and anaerobes
- Specific pediatric dosage guidelines

FOR SIGNIFICANT ECONOMIC REASONS

- Competitively priced
- No price increase since 1984
- May be more cost-effective than combination therapy

See your Merck Representative for a discussion of the potential value of MEFOXIN to your patients and to your hospital.

* Estimate based on total usage in the United States.
† *In vitro* activity does not necessarily imply *in vivo* efficacy.

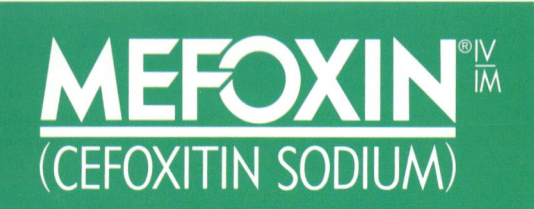

MEFOXIN® IV/IM
(CEFOXITIN SODIUM)

1. Kellum, J.M. et al.: Randomized, prospective comparison of cefoxitin and gentamicin-clindamycin in the treatment of acute colonic diverticulitis, Clin. Ther. *14(3)*:376-384, 1992.
2. Goldstein, E.J.C. and Citron, D.M.: Annual incidence, epidemiology, and comparative in vitro susceptibilities to cefoxitin, cefotetan, cefmetazole, and ceftizoxime of recent community-acquired isolates of the *Bacteroides fragilis* group, J. Clin. Microbiol. *26(11)*:2361-2366, November 1988.
3. Gill, C.J. et al.: In vitro activities of antibacterial agents against clinical isolates of *Escherichia coli* and *Klebsiella* species from intensive care units, Clin. Ther. *13(1)*:25-37, 1991.

...ving full Prescribing Information.

● MERCK

MEFOXIN®
(STERILE CEFOXITIN SODIUM)

MEFOXIN®
(Sterile Cefoxitin Sodium)

DESCRIPTION

MEFOXIN* (Sterile Cefoxitin Sodium) is a semi-synthetic, broad-spectrum cepha antibiotic sealed under nitrogen for parenteral administration. It is derived from cephamycin C, which is produced by *Streptomyces lactamdurans*. It is the sodium salt of 3-(hydroxymethyl)-7α-methoxy-8-oxo-7-[2-(2-thienyl)acetamido]-5-thia-1-azabicyclo [4.2.0] oct-2-ene-2-carboxylate carbamate (ester). The empirical formula is $C_{16}H_{16}N_3NaO_7S_2$, and the structural formula is:

MEFOXIN contains approximately 53.8 mg (2.3 milliequivalents) of sodium per gram of cefoxitin activity. Solutions of MEFOXIN range from colorless to light amber in color. The pH of freshly constituted solutions usually ranges from 4.2 to 7.0.

CLINICAL PHARMACOLOGY

Clinical Pharmacology

After intramuscular administration of a 1 gram dose of MEFOXIN to normal volunteers, the mean peak serum concentration was 24 mcg/mL. The peak occurred at 20 to 30 minutes. Following an intravenous dose of 1 gram, serum concentrations were 110 mcg/mL at 5 minutes, declining to less than 1 mcg/mL at 4 hours. The half-life after an intravenous dose is 41 to 59 minutes; after intramuscular administration, the half-life is 64.8 minutes. Approximately 85 percent of cefoxitin is excreted unchanged by the kidneys over a 6-hour period, resulting in high urinary concentrations. Following an intramuscular dose of 1 gram, urinary concentrations greater than 3000 mcg/mL were observed. Probenecid slows tubular excretion and produces higher serum levels and increases the duration of measurable serum concentrations.

Cefoxitin passes into pleural and joint fluids and is detectable in antibacterial concentrations in bile.

Clinical experience has demonstrated that MEFOXIN can be administered to patients who are also receiving carbenicillin, kanamycin, gentamicin, tobramycin, or amikacin (see PRECAUTIONS and ADMINISTRATION).

Microbiology

The bactericidal action of cefoxitin results from inhibition of cell wall synthesis. Cefoxitin has *in vitro* activity against a wide range of gram-positive and gram-negative organisms. The methoxy group in the 7α position provides MEFOXIN with a high degree of stability in the presence of beta-lactamases, both penicillinases and cephalosporinases, of gram-negative bacteria. Cefoxitin is usually active against the following organisms *in vitro* and in clinical infections:

Gram-positive
  Staphylococcus aureus, including penicillinase and non-penicillinase producing strains

---

*Registered trademark of MERCK & CO., INC.
COPYRIGHT © MERCK & CO., INC., 1985
All rights reserved

MEFOXIN®
(Sterile Cefoxitin Sodium)

  Staphylococcus epidermidis
  Beta-hemolytic and other streptococci (most strains of enterococci, e.g., *Streptococcus faecalis*, are resistant)
  Streptococcus pneumoniae
Gram-negative
  Escherichia coli
  Klebsiella species (including *K. pneumoniae*)
  Hemophilus influenzae
  Neisseria gonorrhoeae, including penicillinase and non-penicillinase producing strains
  Proteus mirabilis
  Morganella morganii
  Proteus vulgaris
  Providencia species, including *Providencia rettgeri*
Anaerobic organisms
  Peptococcus species
  Peptostreptococcus species
  Clostridium species
  Bacteroides species, including the *B. fragilis* group (includes *B. fragilis, B. distasonis, B. ovatus, B. thetaiotaomicron, B. vulgatus*)

MEFOXIN is inactive *in vitro* against most strains of *Pseudomonas aeruginosa* and enterococci and many strains of *Enterobacter cloacae*.

Methicillin-resistant staphylococci are almost uniformly resistant to MEFOXIN.

Susceptibility Tests

For fast-growing aerobic organisms, quantitative methods that require measurements of zone diameters give the most precise estimates of antibiotic susceptibility. One such procedure* has been recommended for use with discs to test susceptibility to cefoxitin. Interpretation involves correlation of the diameters obtained in the disc test with minimal inhibitory concentration (MIC) values for cefoxitin.

Reports from the laboratory giving results of the standardized single disc susceptibility test* using a 30 mcg cefoxitin disc should be interpreted according to the following criteria:

Organisms producing zones of 18 mm or greater are considered susceptible, indicating that the tested organism is likely to respond to therapy.

Organisms of intermediate susceptibility produce zones of 15 to 17 mm, indicating that the tested organism would be susceptible if high dosage is used or if the infection is confined to tissues and fluids (e.g., urine) in which high antibiotic levels are attained.

Resistant organisms produce zones of 14 mm or less, indicating that other therapy should be selected.

The cefoxitin disc should be used for testing cefoxitin susceptibility.

Cefoxitin has been shown by *in vitro* tests to have activity against certain strains of *Enterobacteriaceae* found resistant when tested with the cephalosporin class disc. For this reason, the cefoxitin disc should not be used for testing susceptibility to cephalosporins, and cephalosporin discs should not be used for testing susceptibility to cefoxitin.

Dilution methods, preferably the agar plate dilution procedure, are most accurate for sus-

---

*Bauer, A. W.; Kirby, W. M. M.; Sherris, J. C.; Turck, M.: Antibiotic susceptibility testing by a standardized single disc method, Amer. J. Clin. Path. 45: 493-496, Apr. 1966. Standardized disc susceptibility test, Federal Register 37: 20527-20529, 1972. National Committee for Clinical Laboratory Standards: Approved Standard: ASM-2, Performance Standards for Antimicrobial Disc Susceptibility Tests, July 1975.

MEFOXIN®
(Sterile Cefoxitin Sodium)

ceptibility testing of obligate anaerobes.

A bacterial isolate may be considered susceptible if the MIC value for cefoxitin** is not more than 16 mcg/mL. Organisms are considered resistant if the MIC is greater than 32 mcg/mL.

INDICATIONS AND USAGE

Treatment

MEFOXIN is indicated for the treatment of serious infections caused by susceptible strains of the designated microorganisms in the diseases listed below.

(1) **Lower respiratory tract infections,** including pneumonia and lung abscess, caused by *Streptococcus pneumoniae*, other streptococci (excluding enterococci, e.g., *Streptococcus faecalis*), *Staphylococcus aureus* (penicillinase and non-penicillinase producing), *Escherichia coli*, *Klebsiella* species, *Hemophilus influenzae*, and *Bacteroides* species.

(2) **Genitourinary infections.** Urinary tract infections caused by *Escherichia coli*, *Klebsiella* species, *Proteus mirabilis*, indole-positive Proteus (which include the organisms now called *Morganella morganii* and *Proteus vulgaris*), and *Providencia* species (including *Providencia rettgeri*). Uncomplicated gonorrhea due to *Neisseria gonorrhoeae* (penicillinase and non-penicillinase producing).

(3) **Intra-abdominal infections,** including peritonitis and intra-abdominal abscess, caused by *Escherichia coli*, *Klebsiella* species, *Bacteroides* species including the *Bacteroides fragilis* group*, and *Clostridium* species.

(4) **Gynecological infections,** including endometritis, pelvic cellulitis, and pelvic inflammatory disease caused by *Escherichia coli*, *Neisseria gonorrhoeae* (penicillinase and non-penicillinase producing), *Bacteroides* species including the *Bacteroides fragilis* group*, *Clostridium* species, *Peptococcus* species, *Peptostreptococcus* species, and Group B streptococci.

(5) **Septicemia** caused by *Streptococcus pneumoniae*, *Staphylococcus aureus* (penicillinase and non-penicillinase producing), *Escherichia coli*, *Klebsiella* species, and *Bacteroides* species including the *Bacteroides fragilis* group.*

(6) **Bone and joint infections** caused by *Staphylococcus aureus* (penicillinase and non-penicillinase producing).

(7) **Skin and skin structure infections** caused by *Staphylococcus aureus* (penicillinase and non-penicillinase producing), *Staphylococcus epidermidis*, streptococci (excluding enterococci e.g., *Streptococcus faecalis*), *Escherichia coli*, *Proteus mirabilis*, *Klebsiella* species, *Bacteroides* species including the *Bacteroides fragilis* group*, *Clostridium* species, *Peptococcus* species, and *Peptostreptococcus* species.

Appropriate culture and susceptibility studies should be performed to determine the susceptibility of the causative organisms to MEFOXIN. Therapy may be started while awaiting the results of these studies.

In randomized comparative studies, MEFOXIN and cephalothin were comparably safe and effective in the management of infections caused by gram-positive cocci and gram-negative rods susceptible to the cephalosporins. MEFOXIN has a high degree of stability in the presence of bacterial beta-lactamases, both penicillinases and cephalosporinases.

**B. fragilis, B. distasonis, B. ovatus, B. thetaiotaomicron, B. vulgatus.*

**Determined by the ICS agar dilution method (Ericsson and Sherris, Acta Path. Microbiol. Scand. [B] Suppl. No. 217, 1971) or any other method that has been shown to give equivalent results.

MEFOXIN®
(Sterile Cefoxitin Sodium)

Many infections caused by aerobic and anaerobic gram-negative bacteria resistant to some cephalosporins respond to MEFOXIN. Similarly, many infections caused by aerobic and anaerobic bacteria resistant to some penicillin antibiotics (ampicillin, carbenicillin, penicillin G) respond to treatment with MEFOXIN. Many infections caused by mixtures of susceptible aerobic and anaerobic bacteria respond to treatment with MEFOXIN.

Prevention

When compared to placebo in randomized controlled studies in patients undergoing gastrointestinal surgery, vaginal hysterectomy, abdominal hysterectomy and cesarean section, the prophylactic use of MEFOXIN resulted in a significant reduction in the number of postoperative infections.

The prophylactic administration of MEFOXIN may reduce the incidence of certain postoperative infections in patients undergoing surgical procedures (e.g., hysterectomy, gastrointestinal surgery and transurethral prostatectomy) that are classified as contaminated or potentially contaminated.

The perioperative use of MEFOXIN may be effective in surgical patients in whom subsequent infection at the operative site would present a serious risk, e.g., prosthetic arthroplasty.

Effective prophylactic use depends on the time of administration. MEFOXIN usually should be given one-half to one hour before the operation, which is sufficient time to achieve effective levels in the wound during the procedure. Prophylactic administration should usually be stopped within 24 hours since continuing administration of any antibiotic increases the possibility of adverse reactions but, in the majority of surgical procedures, does not reduce the incidence of subsequent infection. However, in patients undergoing prosthetic arthroplasty, it is recommended that MEFOXIN be continued for 72 hours after the surgical procedure.

If there are signs of infection, specimens for culture should be obtained for identification of the causative organism so that appropriate treatment may be instituted.

CONTRAINDICATIONS

MEFOXIN is contraindicated in patients who have shown hypersensitivity to cefoxitin and the cephalosporin group of antibiotics.

WARNINGS

BEFORE THERAPY WITH 'MEFOXIN' IS INSTITUTED, CAREFUL INQUIRY SHOULD BE MADE TO DETERMINE WHETHER THE PATIENT HAS HAD PREVIOUS HYPERSENSITIVITY REACTIONS TO CEFOXITIN, CEPHALOSPORINS, PENICILLINS, OR OTHER DRUGS. THIS PRODUCT SHOULD BE GIVEN WITH CAUTION TO PENICILLIN-SENSITIVE PATIENTS. ANTIBIOTICS SHOULD BE ADMINISTERED WITH CAUTION TO ANY PATIENT WHO HAS DEMONSTRATED SOME FORM OF ALLERGY, PARTICULARLY TO DRUGS. IF AN ALLERGIC REACTION TO 'MEFOXIN' OCCURS, DISCONTINUE THE DRUG. SERIOUS HYPERSENSITIVITY REACTIONS MAY REQUIRE EPINEPHRINE AND OTHER EMERGENCY MEASURES.

Pseudomembranous colitis has been reported with virtually all antibiotics (including

MEFOXIN®
(Sterile Cefoxitin Sodium)

cephalosporins); therefore, it is important to consider its diagnosis in patients who develop diarrhea in association with antibiotic use. This colitis may range from mild to life threatening in severity.

Treatment with broad-spectrum antibiotics alters normal flora of the colon and may permit overgrowth of clostridia. Studies indicate a toxin produced by *clostridium difficile* is one primary cause of antibiotic-associated colitis.

Mild cases of pseudomembranous colitis may respond to drug discontinuance alone. In more severe cases, management may include sigmoidoscopy, appropriate bacteriological studies, fluid, electrolyte and protein supplementation, and the use of a drug such as oral vancomycin as indicated. Isolation of the patient may be advisable. Other causes of colitis should also be considered.

PRECAUTIONS

General

The total daily dose should be reduced when MEFOXIN is administered to patients with transient or persistent reduction of urinary output due to renal insufficiency (see DOSAGE), because high and prolonged serum antibiotic concentrations can occur in such individuals from usual doses.

Antibiotics (including cephalosporins) should be prescribed with caution in individuals with a history of gastrointestinal disease, particularly colitis.

As with other antibiotics, prolonged use of MEFOXIN may result in overgrowth of nonsusceptible organisms. Repeated evaluation of the patient's condition is essential. If superinfection occurs during therapy, appropriate measures should be taken.

Drug Interactions

Increased nephrotoxicity has been reported following concomitant administration of cephalosporins and aminoglycoside antibiotics.

Drug/Laboratory Test Interactions

As with cephalothin, high concentrations of cefoxitin (>100 micrograms/mL) may interfere with measurement of serum and urine creatinine levels by the Jaffé reaction, and produce false increases of modest degree in the levels of creatinine reported. Serum samples from patients treated with cefoxitin should not be analyzed for creatinine if withdrawn within 2 hours of drug administration.

High concentrations of cefoxitin in the urine may interfere with measurement of urinary 17-hydroxy-corticosteroids by the Porter-Silber reaction, and produce false increases of modest degree in the levels reported.

A false-positive reaction for glucose in the urine may occur. This has been observed with CLINITEST* reagent tablets.

Carcinogenesis, Mutagenesis, Impairment of Fertility

Long-term studies in animals have not been performed with cefoxitin to evaluate carcinogenic or mutagenic potential. Studies in rats treated intravenously with 400 mg/kg of cefoxitin (approximately three times the maximum recommended human dose) revealed no effects on fertility or mating ability.

Pregnancy

Pregnancy Category B. Reproduction studies performed in rats and mice at parenteral doses of approximately one to seven and one-half times the maximum recommended human dose did not reveal teratogenic or fetal toxic effects, although a slight decrease in fetal weight was observed.

---

*Registered trademark of Ames Company, Division of Miles Laboratories, Inc.

MEFOXIN®
(Sterile Cefoxitin Sodium)

There are, however, no adequate and well-controlled studies in pregnant women. Because animal reproduction studies are not always predictive of human response, this drug should be used during pregnancy only if clearly needed.

In the rabbit, cefoxitin was associated with a high incidence of abortion and maternal death. This was not considered to be a teratogenic effect but an expected consequence of the rabbit's unusual sensitivity to antibiotic-induced changes in the population of the microflora of the intestine.

Nursing Mothers

MEFOXIN is excreted in human milk in low concentrations. Caution should be exercised when MEFOXIN is administered to a nursing woman.

Pediatric Use

Safety and efficacy in infants from birth to three months of age have not yet been established. In children three months of age and older, higher doses of MEFOXIN have been associated with an increased incidence of eosinophilia and elevated SGOT.

ADVERSE REACTIONS

MEFOXIN is generally well tolerated. The most common adverse reactions have been local reactions following intravenous or intramuscular injection. Other adverse reactions have been encountered infrequently.

Local Reactions

Thrombophlebitis has occurred with intravenous administration. Pain, induration, and tenderness after intramuscular injections have been reported.

Allergic Reactions

Rash (including exfoliative dermatitis), pruritus, eosinophilia, fever, dyspnea, and other allergic reactions including anaphylaxis and angioedema have been noted.

Cardiovascular

Hypotension

Gastrointestinal

Diarrhea, including documented pseudomembranous colitis which can appear during or after antibiotic treatment. Nausea and vomiting have been reported rarely.

Blood

Eosinophilia, leukopenia including granulocytopenia, neutropenia, anemia, including hemolytic anemia, thrombocytopenia, and bone marrow depression. A positive direct Coombs test may develop in some individuals, especially those with azotemia.

Liver Function

Transient elevations in SGOT, SGPT, serum LDH, and serum alkaline phosphatase; and jaundice have been reported.

Renal Function

Elevations in serum creatinine and/or blood urea nitrogen levels have been observed. As with the cephalosporins, acute renal failure has been reported rarely. The role of MEFOXIN in changes in renal function tests is difficult to assess, since factors predisposing to prerenal azotemia or to impaired renal function usually have been present.

OVERDOSAGE

The acute intravenous LD_{50} in the adult female mouse and rabbit was about 8.0 g/kg and greater than 1.0 g/kg respectively. The acute intraperitoneal LD_{50} in the adult rat was greater than 10.0 g/kg.

DOSAGE

TREATMENT

Adults

The usual adult dosage range is 1 gram to 2

MEFOXIN®
(Sterile Cefoxitin Sodium)

grams every six to eight hours. Dosage and route of administration should be determined by susceptibility of the causative organisms, severity of infection, and the condition of the patient (see Table 1 for dosage guidelines).

MEFOXIN may be used in patients with reduced renal function with the following dosage adjustments:

In adults with renal insufficiency, an initial loading dose of 1 gram to 2 grams may be given. After a loading dose, the recommendations for *maintenance dosage* (Table 2) may be used as a guide.

When only the serum creatinine level is available, the following formula (based on sex, weight, and age of the patient) may be used to convert this value into creatinine clearance. The serum creatinine should represent a steady state of renal function.

Males: $\dfrac{\text{Weight (kg)} \times (140 - \text{age})}{72 \times \text{serum creatinine (mg/100 mL)}}$

Females: 0.85 × above value

In patients undergoing hemodialysis, the loading dose of 1 to 2 grams should be given after each hemodialysis, and the maintenance dose should be given as indicated in Table 2.

Antibiotic therapy for group A beta-hemolytic streptococcal infections should be maintained for at least 10 days to guard against the risk of rheumatic fever or glomerulonephritis. In staphylococcal and other infections involving a collection of pus, surgical drainage should be carried out where indicated.

The recommended dosage of MEFOXIN for **uncomplicated gonorrhea** is 2 grams intramuscularly, with 1 gram of BENEMID* (Probenecid) given by mouth at the same time or up to ½ hour before MEFOXIN.

Infants and Children

The recommended dosage in children three months of age and older is 80 to 160 mg/kg of body weight per day divided into four to six equal doses. The higher dosages should be used for more severe or serious infections. The total daily dosage should not exceed 12 grams.

At this time no recommendation is made for children from birth to three months of age (see PRECAUTIONS).

In children with renal insufficiency the dosage and frequency of dosage should be modified consistent with the recommendations for adults (see Table 2).

PREVENTION
General

For prophylactic use in surgery, the following doses are recommended:

Adults:
(1) 2 grams administered intravenously or intramuscularly just prior to surgery (approximately one-half to one hour before the initial incision).
(2) 2 grams every 6 hours after the first dose for no more than 24 hours (continued for 72 hours after prosthetic arthroplasty).

Children (3 months and older):
30 to 40 mg/kg doses may be given at the times designated above.

Obstetric-Gynecologic

For prophylactic use in vaginal hysterectomy, a single 2.0 gram dose administered intramuscularly one-half to one hour prior to surgery is recommended.

For patients undergoing cesarean section, a single 2.0 gram dose should be administered intravenously as soon as the umbilical cord is clamped. A 3-dose regimen may be more effective than a single dose regimen in preventing postoperative infection (esp. endometritis) following cesarean section. Such a regimen would consist of 2.0 grams given intravenously as soon as the umbilical cord is clamped, followed by 2.0 grams 4 and 8 hours after the initial dose.

Transurethral prostatectomy patients:

One gram administered just prior to surgery; 1 gram every 8 hours for up to five days.

Table 1 — Guidelines for Dosage of MEFOXIN

Type of Infection	Daily Dosage	Frequency and Route
Uncomplicated forms+ of infections such as pneumonia, urinary tract infection, cutaneous infection	3 - 4 grams	1 gram every 6 - 8 hours IV or IM
Moderately severe or severe infections	6 - 8 grams	1 gram every 4 hours *or* 2 grams every 6 - 8 hours IV
Infections commonly needing antibiotics in higher dosage (e.g., gas gangrene)	12 grams	2 grams every 4 hours *or* 3 grams every 6 hours IV

+Including patients in whom bacteremia is absent or unlikely.

Table 2 — Maintenance Dosage of MEFOXIN in Adults with Reduced Renal Function

Renal Function	Creatinine Clearance (mL/min)	Dose (grams)	Frequency
Mild impairment	50 - 30	1 - 2	every 8 - 12 hours
Moderate impairment	29 - 10	1 - 2	every 12 - 24 hours
Severe impairment	9 - 5	0.5 - 1	every 12 - 24 hours
Essentially no function	< 5	0.5 - 1	every 24 - 48 hours

Table 3 — Preparation of Solution

Strength	Amount of Diluent to be Added (mL)++	Approximate Withdrawable Volume (mL)	Approximate Average Concentration (mg/mL)
1 gram Vial	2 (Intramuscular)	2.5	400
2 gram Vial	4 (Intramuscular)	5	400
1 gram Vial	10 (IV)	10.5	95
2 gram Vial	10 or 20 (IV)	11.1 or 21.0	180 or 95
1 gram Infusion Bottle	50 or 100 (IV)	50 or 100	20 or 10
2 gram Infusion Bottle	50 or 100 (IV)	50 or 100	40 or 20
10 gram Bulk	43 or 93 (IV)	49 or 98.5	200 or 100

++Shake to dissolve and let stand until clear.

*Registered trademark of MERCK & CO., INC.

MEFOXIN®
(Sterile Cefoxitin Sodium)

PREPARATION OF SOLUTION

Table 3 is provided for convenience in constituting MEFOXIN for both intravenous and intramuscular administration.

For intravenous use, 1 gram should be constituted with at least 10 mL of Sterile Water for Injection, and 2 grams, with 10 or 20 mL. The 10 gram bulk package should be constituted with 43 or 93 mL of Sterile Water for Injection or any of the solutions listed under the *Intravenous* portion of the COMPATIBILITY AND STABILITY section. CAUTION: THE 10 GRAM BULK STOCK SOLUTION IS NOT FOR DIRECT INFUSION. One or 2 grams of MEFOXIN for infusion may be constituted with 50 or 100 mL of 0.9 percent Sodium Chloride Injection, 5 percent or 10 percent Dextrose Injection, or any of the solutions listed under the *Intravenous* portion of the COMPATIBILITY AND STABILITY section.

Benzyl alcohol as a preservative has been associated with toxicity in neonates. While toxicity has not been demonstrated in infants greater than three months of age, in whom use of MEFOXIN may be indicated, small infants in this age range may also be at risk for benzyl alcohol toxicity. Therefore, diluent containing benzyl alcohol should not be used when MEFOXIN is constituted for administration to infants.

For ADD-Vantage®* vials, see separate INSTRUCTIONS FOR USE OF MEFOXIN IN ADD-Vantage® VIALS. MEFOXIN in ADD-Vantage® vials should be constituted with ADD-Vantage® diluent containers containing 50 mL or 100 mL of either 0.9 percent Sodium Chloride Injection or 5 percent Dextrose Injection. MEFOXIN in ADD-Vantage® vials is for IV use only.

For intramuscular use, each gram of MEFOXIN may be constituted with 2 mL of Sterile Water for Injection, *or—*

For intramuscular use ONLY: each gram of MEFOXIN may be constituted with 2 mL of 0.5 percent lidocaine hydrochloride solution† (without epinephrine) to minimize the discomfort of intramuscular injection.

ADMINISTRATION

MEFOXIN may be administered intravenously or intramuscularly after constitution.

Parenteral drug products should be inspected visually for particulate matter and discoloration prior to administration whenever solution and container permit.

Intravenous Administration

The intravenous route is preferable for patients with bacteremia, bacterial septicemia, or other severe or life-threatening infections, or for patients who may be poor risks because of lowered resistance resulting from such debilitating conditions as malnutrition, trauma, surgery, diabetes, heart failure, or malignancy, particularly if shock is present or impending.

For intermittent intravenous administration, a solution containing 1 gram or 2 grams in 10 mL of Sterile Water for Injection can be injected over a period of three to five minutes. Using an infusion system, it may also be given over a longer period of time through the tubing system by which the patient may be receiving other intravenous solutions. However, during infusion of the solution containing MEFOXIN, it is advisable to temporarily discontinue administration of any other solutions at the same site.

---
*Registered trademark of Abbott Laboratories, Inc.
†See package circular of manufacturer for detailed information concerning contraindications, warnings, precautions, and adverse reactions.

MEFOXIN®
(Sterile Cefoxitin Sodium)

For the administration of higher doses by continuous intravenous infusion, a solution of MEFOXIN may be added to an intravenous bottle containing 5 percent Dextrose Injection, 0.9 percent Sodium Chloride Injection, 5 percent Dextrose and 0.9 percent Sodium Chloride Injection, or 5 percent Dextrose Injection with 0.02 percent sodium bicarbonate solution. BUTTERFLY* or scalp vein-type needles are preferred for this type of infusion.

Solutions of MEFOXIN, like those of most beta-lactam antibiotics, should not be added to aminoglycoside solutions (e.g., gentamicin sulfate, tobramycin sulfate, amikacin sulfate) because of potential interaction. However, MEFOXIN and aminoglycosides may be administered separately to the same patient.

Intramuscular Administration

As with all intramuscular preparations, MEFOXIN should be injected well within the body of a relatively large muscle such as the upper outer quadrant of the buttock (i.e., gluteus maximus); aspiration is necessary to avoid inadvertent injection into a blood vessel.

COMPATIBILITY AND STABILITY

Intravenous

MEFOXIN, as supplied in vials or the bulk package and constituted to 1 gram/10 mL with Sterile Water for Injection, Bacteriostatic Water for Injection, (see PREPARATION OF SOLUTION), 0.9 percent Sodium Chloride Injection, or 5 percent Dextrose Injection, maintains satisfactory potency for 24 hours at room temperature, for one week under refrigeration (below 5°C), and for at least 30 weeks in the frozen state.

These primary solutions may be further diluted in 50 to 1000 mL of the following solutions and maintain potency for 24 hours at room temperature and at least 48 hours under refrigeration:

Sterile Water for Injection‡
0.9 percent Sodium Chloride Injection
5 percent or 10 percent Dextrose Injection‡
5 percent Dextrose and 0.9 percent Sodium Chloride Injection
5 percent Dextrose Injection with 0.02 percent Sodium Bicarbonate solution
5 percent Dextrose Injection with 0.2 percent or 0.45 percent saline solution
Ringer's Injection
Lactated Ringer's Injection‡
5 percent Dextrose in Lactated Ringer's Injection‡
5 percent or 10 percent invert sugar in water
10 percent invert sugar in saline solution
5 percent Sodium Bicarbonate Injection
Neut (sodium bicarbonate)*‡
M/6 sodium lactate solution
NORMOSOL-M in D5-W*‡
IONOSOL B w/Dextrose 5 percent*‡
POLYONIC M 56 in 5 percent Dextrose**
Mannitol 5% and 2.5%
Mannitol 10%‡
ISOLYTE*** E
ISOLYTE*** E with 5% Dextrose

MEFOXIN, as supplied in infusion bottles and constituted with 50 to 100 mL of 0.9 percent Sodium Chloride Injection, or 5 percent or 10 percent Dextrose Injection, maintains satisfac-

---
*Registered trademark of Abbott Laboratories, Inc.
‡In these solutions, MEFOXIN has been found to be stable for a period of one week under refrigeration.
**Registered trademark of Cutter Laboratories, Inc.
***Registered trademark of American Hospital Supply Corporation.

MEFOXIN®
(Sterile Cefoxitin Sodium)

tory potency for 24 hours at room temperature or for 1 week under refrigeration (below 5°C).

MEFOXIN is supplied in single dose ADD-Vantage® vials and should be prepared as directed in the accompanying INSTRUCTIONS FOR USE OF MEFOXIN IN ADD-Vantage® VIALS using ADD-Vantage® diluent containers containing 50 mL or 100 mL of either 0.9 percent Sodium Chloride Injection or 5 percent Dextrose Injection. When prepared with either of these diluents, MEFOXIN maintains satisfactory potency for 24 hours at room temperature.

Limited studies with solutions of MEFOXIN in 0.9 percent Sodium Chloride Injection, Lactated Ringer's Injection, and 5 percent Dextrose Injection in VIAFLEX† intravenous bags show stability for 24 hours at room temperature, 48 hours under refrigeration or 26 weeks in the frozen state and 24 hours at room temperature thereafter. Also, solutions of MEFOXIN in 0.9 percent Sodium Chloride Injection show similar stability in plastic tubing, drip chambers, and volume control devices of common intravenous infusion sets.

After constitution with Sterile Water for Injection and subsequent storage in disposable plastic syringes, MEFOXIN is stable for 24 hours at room temperature and 48 hours under refrigeration.

After the periods mentioned above, any unused solutions or frozen material should be discarded. Do not refreeze.

Intramuscular
MEFOXIN, as constituted with Sterile Water for Injection, Bacteriostatic Water for Injection, or 0.5 percent or 1 percent lidocaine hydrochloride solution (without epinephrine), maintains satisfactory potency for 24 hours at room temperature, for one week under refrigeration (below 5°C), and for at least 30 weeks in the frozen state.

After the periods mentioned above, any unused solutions or frozen material should be discarded. Do not refreeze.

MEFOXIN has also been found compatible when admixed in intravenous infusions with the following:

Heparin 0.1 units/mL at room temperature — 8 hours

Heparin 100 units/mL at room temperature — 24 hours

M.V.I.†† concentrate at room temperature 24 hours; under refrigeration 48 hours

BEROCCA††† C-500 at room temperature 24 hours; under refrigeration 48 hours

†Registered trademark of Baxter International, Inc.
††Registered trademark of USV Pharmaceutical Corp.
†††Registered trademark of Roche Laboratories.

MEFOXIN®
(Sterile Cefoxitin Sodium)

Insulin in Normal Saline at room temperature 24 hours; under refrigeration 48 hours

Insulin in 10% invert sugar at room temperature 24 hours; under refrigeration 48 hours

HOW SUPPLIED

Sterile MEFOXIN is a dry white to off-white powder supplied in vials and infusion bottles containing cefoxitin sodium as follows:

No. 3356 — 1 gram cefoxitin equivalent
NDC 0006-3356-45 in trays of 25 vials
(6505-01-119-6005, 1 g 25's).

No. 3368 — 1 gram cefoxitin equivalent
NDC 0006-3368-71 in trays of 10 infusion bottles
(6505-01-195-0649, 1 g infusion bottle 10's).

No. 3357 — 2 gram cefoxitin equivalent
NDC 0006-3357-53 in trays of 25 vials
(6505-01-104-6393, 2 g 25's).

No. 3369 — 2 gram cefoxitin equivalent
NDC 0006-3369-73 in trays of 10 infusion bottles
(6505-01-185-2624, 2 g infusion bottle 10's).

No. 3388 — 10 gram cefoxitin equivalent
NDC 0006-3388-67 in trays of 6 bulk bottles
(6505-01-263-0730, 10 g 6's).

No. 3548 — 1 gram cefoxitin equivalent
NDC 0006-3548-45 in trays of 25 ADD-Vantage® vials
(6505-01-262-9509, 1 g ADD-Vantage® 25's).

No. 3549 — 2 gram cefoxitin equivalent
NDC 0006-3549-53 in trays of 25 ADD-Vantage® vials
(6505-01-263-4531, 2 g ADD-Vantage® 25's).

Special storage instructions
MEFOXIN in the dry state should be stored below 30°C. Avoid exposure to temperatures above 50°C. The dry material as well as solutions tend to darken, depending on storage conditions; product potency, however, is not adversely affected.

MERCK SHARP & DOHME, Division of Merck & Co., INC.
West Point, Pa. 19486

A.H.F.S. Category: 8:12.07

Issued January 1992

DC7057130